An Introduction to Evidence-based Practice in Nursing & Healthcare

Dr. Alison Pooler

WITHDRAWN

Harlow, England • London • New York • Boston • San Francisco • Toronto
Sydney • Tokyo • Singapore • Hong Kong • Seoul • Taipei • New Delhi
Cape Town • Madrid • Mexico City • Amsterdam • Munich • Paris • Milan

Pearson Education Limited
Edinburgh Gate
Harlow
Essex CM20 2JE
England

and Associated Companies throughout the world

Visit us on the World Wide Web at:
www.pearsoned.co.uk

First published 2011

© Pearson Education Limited 2012

ISBN: 978-0-273-72295-3

British Library Cataloguing-in-Publication Data
A catalogue record for this book is available from the British Library

Library of Congress Cataloging-in-Publication Data
Pooler, Alison.
    An introduction to evidence-based practice in nursing and healthcare / Alison Pooler.
        p. ; cm.
    Includes bibliographical references and index.
    ISBN 978-0-273-72295-3 (pbk.)
1. Evidence-based medicine. I. Title.
    [DNLM: 1. Evidence-Based Practice. WB 102.5]
    R723.7.P66 2012
    610.73--dc23

                                                                    2011022071

10 9 8 7 6 5 4 3 2 1
15 14 13 12 11

Typeset in 9.5/12.5pt Interstate Light by 35
Printed and bound in Malaysia (CTP-VVP)

Contents

Preface

The understanding and application of evidence base to clinical practice is embedded in all areas of healthcare. Seeking an evidence base for what we do in practice is not a new concept, but one which has had intense focus on over the past decade from the government and their drive for improved quality in healthcare and accountability. It is now at the forefront of healthcare and a concept that is central to the education and training of healthcare professionals.

This book is designed to help students to gain a basic understanding of the area of evidence-based practice. Many books presume an understanding of some of the basic principles and concepts and, unless these are understood, then the study of evidence-based practice is impeded. This book begins with definitions of what evidence-based practice is, what research is and how we find it. What do we do with research once we have found it and then how do we apply it to practice? Applying evidence to practice is not easy and involves change, which again is a challenging concept. Some basic principles of change management are discussed at the end of the book. This book provides a stepping stone for the student to move next on to a more advanced text in the subject area.

A. Pooler 2011

Chapter 1

What is research?

AIMS

When you have read this chapter, you should understand:

- The definition of what research is
- The different methodologies employed within research
- The positive and negative aspects of the research methodologies

Introduction

A tutor stood in front of a class and asked the students what they understood by the term 'research'. A variety of responses came back, which included 'research is about looking at the literature on a topic area and deciding what is best', 'it is about experiments' and 'it's all about publishing papers'.

From this the tutor is able to see that there is a diverse range in the understanding and misunderstanding of the term research. This case highlights the importance of gaining a basic and accurate understanding of what research actually is before we can continue on with this book.

ACTIVITY 1.1

Before you go any further, write down your answer to 'what is research?' Keep this definition handy and then review it again when you have finished reading this chapter to see if it has changed or not.

....

....

....

....

What is research?

It is now widely accepted that all healthcare professionals need to be aware of and be knowledgeable about what research is and the application of the research process and outcomes to their own clinical areas. Research has become a commonly used term in our professional vocabulary and it is expected that all healthcare professionals gain familiarity with research and its appropriate use. So what is research?

The essential nature of research lies in its intent to create new knowledge in whatever field' (Cormack et al., 2006: p. ,93). It achieves this through a process and is guided by scientific principles, depending on the area in which the research is carried out and the methodology used.

Research can also be defined as a search for knowledge, or a systematic investigation to establish facts. The primary purpose of research may be to discover, interpret and develop methods and systems for the advancement of human knowledge on a wide variety of subject matters. In health and healthcare, this can range from a randomised controlled double-blinded study on the effect of a new drug to discovering patients' feelings of an element of their care to the evaluation of the cost-effectiveness of a patient-led service and the clinical and economic outcome. The areas of research are immense and many different methodologies, which will be classified later, are used.

Generally, research is understood to follow a certain structural process. Although step order may vary depending on the subject matter, the following steps are usually part of most formal research.

- Formation of the topic area
- Defining the hypothesis – an idea of what the question/answer may be that you are trying to find out
- Justification of why the research needs to be done, through a review of the literature in the topic area
- Defining the methodology
- Pilot study
- Redefining, if necessary, following the pilot study
- Gathering of data
- Analysis of data
- Discussion of the results generated from the analysis of the data
- Recommendations to clinical practice and future research.

So, let us go back to the case study at the start of this section. If the tutor again asked the question 'what is research?' to his group, hopefully the students, now with increased knowledge and awareness of the subject, would answer 'it is a process of advancing knowledge in a certain subject area', 'it is about answering an unknown question', 'it is about discovering new facts and concepts to help in the advancement of healthcare' and 'it helps to ensure that we give the best care to our patients'.

What was the answer that you wrote down at the start of this chapter?

Research methodologies

Now that we understand what research is, we need to start to understand the different methodologies, or ways, of conducting the research. Two very broad methods used in carrying out research are qualitative and quantitative research. We will start by understanding what qualitative research is and then contrast this to what quantitative research is. By doing this, we will see that each methodology has its good points and bad points. These need to be considered when undertaking a research project and also taken into account when you are reading a paper and evaluating its value.

Qualitative research

Qualitative research aims to gather an in-depth understanding of human behaviour and the factors that govern such behaviour. This is very relevant to healthcare, but is also a methodology commonly used in the social sciences and market research. When I say that qualitative research looks at human behaviour, it investigates the 'why' and 'how' of decision-making, not just the 'what', 'where' and 'when'.

Let's take, for example, a ward sister wanting to evaluate whether the method of admitting the patient onto the ward is effective. She would devise a set of questions that are both open-ended and closed so that she could get responses back from the patients and the staff about their thoughts and feelings on what worked well and what did not. The information would be narrative, i.e. words, stories and discussions, and it would be very descriptive, rather than a page of numbers, which is what quantitative research is all about.

Another example may be that a hospital manager wanted to gain insight into whether the nurses that she had put through a nurse prescribing course were using their new skills effectively in practice. Again, questions would be asked, and verbal or written free text would be collected, which would provide a wealth of in-depth context and understanding into the area.

Qualitative research, because of its nature, does not need a large number of participants in the study, which is where it differs from quantitative research. Very often the study groups are small and focused, i.e. they are chosen to take part in the study because of who they are, or what needs they have because of their health condition. This is referred to as purposive sampling.

Types of qualitative research

There are some specific approaches to qualitative research that deserve a mention here, so that you will understand the different ways in which this type of research is carried out, and what these common terms mean when you come across them. If you gain an insight into these different approaches you will then understand why one approach may be selected to answer a specific research question.

1. *Grounded theory*: this is one of the first qualitative research approaches, and was developed by Glaser and Straus in 1967 (Glaser and Straus, 1999). The purpose of this approach is systematically to develop a theory from a set of data that are collected for the purpose of the specific research question under study. The data is usually collected through interviews and observations.

2. *Phenomenology*: this is the study of the lived experience. It is the study of 'phenomena' – the appearances of things and the meanings they have in our experience. In a phenomenological study, the research topic is studied from the point of view of the lived experience of the research participant. Data is usually collected through in-depth interviews, which allow the participant to explore and give a full account of the lived experience.

3. *Ethnography*: this is the study of human social phenomena or culture. This type of research focuses on a community to gain insight about how its members behave. Participant observation and/or in-depth interviews may be used to gain the data for the study. The researchers in ethnographic studies usually carry out first-hand observation of daily behaviour, e.g. observing how healthcare professionals act in a hospital setting. They may even participate in the actual process as a participant observer. This is a

very time-consuming form of research, but results in a real insight into a situation from being part of that situation or environment.

4. *Action research*: this is the process where practitioners attempt to study their problems scientifically to guide, correct and evaluate their decisions and actions. Action research is often designed and conducted by practitioners, who analyse the data to improve their own practice, and is therefore very common in healthcare. The outcome of action research is that it has the potential to generate genuine and sustained improvements in organisations because they have been involved in the process and research has not been imposed on them from research performed outside the organisation.

Qualitative research is a term that encompasses many methodologies and with this come many ways of collecting the data which are employed in these methodologies. These can include:

● Focus groups
● Surveys and **questionnaires**
● Participant observation
● Interviewing.

Very often the data gathered from interviews is recorded and later transcribed. Qualitative research gathers non-numerical data, and this is the big difference between qualitative and quantitative research. It is more about descriptions, themes and an understanding of the workings of a situation. It focuses on language, signs and meanings, and is more holistic and contextual.

One aspect of qualitative research, for which it is sometimes criticised, is the position of the researcher in the process of conducting the research. There is always the fear of the study being **biased** or falsely interpreted by the researcher, which would make it invalid and worthless. The researcher has to try and remain neutral about the area that they are investigating. For example, if a study involved asking patients to write down their thoughts and feelings of the service they had received from a certain clinic, it would be important that they were not aided in the completion of the questions by a researcher who was a member of staff from that clinic. Such a researcher could influence the patients in their response to the questions and encourage their own views to be swayed. A total waste of time and money and no positive outcome would be achieved from the whole process.

There is also the fact that people may behave differently if they know they are being observed or asked about something, especially if the person doing the asking is linked to that area. For example, if the ward sister asks for feedback on the patient's stay on the ward, she may get a biased response rather than if someone separate from the ward asks the same questions, especially if the patient has to come back to that area for a clinic appointment. This is called the **Hawthorne effect**.

Analysing qualitative data

Once data has been collected in a qualitative study, there are various ways of analysing it. Most of the approaches involve transcribing recorded interviews, assigning a code to each section of the transcribed data and then ordering (making sense of) these codes to form categories or themes. These categories or themes are then used to build a description of the results.

It is important that when researchers analyse the data, they do not impose their own preconceived ideas onto the dataset. They do not set out looking for specific ideas, hoping to confirm pre-existing beliefs. Instead, data is coded according to ideas arising from within it. This process is often referred to as inductive.

Methods of maintaining unbiased data analysis include having other people to code and analyse the data, either someone completely uninvolved with the researcher or as a secondary analysis to the researcher who has done the primary analysis. This ensures the quality and rigor of the data produced and maintains objectivity as far as possible.

Quantitative research

Quantitative research is very different from qualitative research in that it uses experimental methods and methods that involve the use of numbers in the collection of data. It is focused on the topic area under study and can sometimes focus on a very small part of a complete area. In healthcare, quantitative methods can sometimes be referred to as clinical trials, where two treatment groups are compared and the outcome measured in numerical terms. Very often a **control group** is used; for example, in many drug trials one group of participants is given the actual drug under study and the other group, the control group, is given a **placebo** and the effects and outcomes are measured and compared.

The principal aim of quantitative research, whatever method is employed, is to seek causal determination and predictability of whether something is true or if something will happen because of something else or by chance. Quantitative data is numerical and is analysed using statistical methods and tests.

Because relationships need to be proven and the occurrence of something happening by chance eliminated, there often needs to be a larger number of participants in the study than would be the case for qualitative research. This is so the findings can be applied in other contexts and chance has been eliminated. Very often the researcher is detached from the study situation and only records the data, rather than being integrally involved as in some qualitative studies.

Types of quantitative research

There are various methodologies employed in quantitative research and these include the following.

1. *Randomised controlled trials*: these are a form of clinical trial and are used to determine the effectiveness of a treatment/ medicine or intervention; for example, if a certain drug has a positive effect on a certain disease process or if attending a specific clinic has an effect on the wellbeing of that patient. Randomised controlled trials are considered to be the highest quality in terms of producing **valid** results and often termed the 'gold standard'. The methods used are very strict and stringent, such as participants being randomly allocated to treatment groups (called randomisation) and the use of placebos. Sometimes not even the researcher has any control over which participant goes into which group or, in the case of a drug trial, who will have the placebos. This is called blinding. Obviously, there are a lot of ethical considerations in randomised controlled trials, especially with the use of placebos. It is only ethical if, by not treating a group, they will not come to any harm. **Informed consent** also needs to be received from any participant involved in a clinical trial.

For example, a consultant wanted to assess the effectiveness of adding in a long-acting bronchodilator to patients already taking a high dose of inhaled steroid. He gathered together all the patients who fitted the inclusion criteria for this trial, depending on their level of inhaled medication and a diagnosis of asthma. All the patients were given a number and were then randomly allocated to either group 1 or group 2.

The pharmacy department made up some inhalers where batch 1 had the steroid in that the patients were already using and batch 2 contained the steroid and an extra drug, the long-acting bronchodilator. The inhalers looked identical and the pharmacy technician was the only person who knew which were which. This is called double blinding as neither the participant nor the researcher (the consultant) knows which are the true inhalers and which are the placebos.

Group 1 were given batch 1 of inhalers and group 2 were given batch 2 of inhalers. They were all monitored with a record of their lung function and symptoms for a period of time and then the results were compared. All the numerical data gathered about the patients' asthma control were entered into a statistical software package and analysed. The results showed that the group with the added long-acting bronchodilator had better lung function and fewer symptoms in comparison with the other group. This showed the benefit of adding in this drug. The study was unbiased because no one other than the pharmacy technician knew which inhalers were which and the participants were randomly allocated to the two groups.

2. *Cohort or case studies*: these are observational studies. You may say that qualitative research involves observation of study participants, but the difference comes from the data generated. In **cohort** or case **studies**, the data is numerical, not narratives or descriptions as in qualitative research. These methodologies attempt to discover links between different factors and are used

when it is not possible to carry out a controlled trial. They are often used to find causes of diseases or to monitor the effects of health activities. The following is an example of a cohort study because everyone in the study is exposed to a particular event or lifestyle; for example, they may all be smokers or all have diabetes that is controlled with insulin.

One of the most famous cohort studies was carried out by Doll and Hill in 1954, where they followed up a group of doctors, some of whom smoked and some did not (Doll *et al.*, 2004). They saw from their observations that those who smoked were more likely to develop lung cancer.

A case study is where patients with a particular condition are studied and compared with others who do not have the condition. This is to try and establish what has caused the condition in the first place.

You can see why different methodologies are employed. A randomised controlled trial would not have been suitable for Doll and Hill's study because it would have been unethical to take one group of people and ask them to smoke so that you could compare them to a group who didn't smoke, all to see if they developed lung cancer!

As you can imagine, these sorts of methodologies require large numbers of study participants and also take a long time to undertake, many years in some cases. Very often questionnaires are used to gather the data, which is numerical and is analysed using statistical methods.

3. *Cross-sectional studies/surveys*: this is where a sample is taken at a given point in time from a predefined population and observed and/or assessed, e.g. asking shoppers at Tesco what they think about something or asking a group of patients waiting in the outpatients department on a certain day about something. Data is usually collected by the use of questionnaires or surveys, which are a predetermined list of questions used to find out specific information about the study subject matter. The quality of the information gained is determined by the quality of the questionnaires used, and care has to be given to the development of the questions to ensure that they are not leading and that they will extract the information required.

The purpose of a cross-sectional study is to provide a snapshot insight into a given population that is under study. For example, a cross-sectional study could be carried out by asking the patients at a GP's surgery about the service they receive, and highlighting different aspects that they need to answer questions on (such as waiting time, comfort, helpfulness of staff, availability of appointments, etc.). The questions are very specific and the patients attending the surgery on the day of the survey should be a representative group of the surgery population as a whole. The information gained would be helpful in developing the service to patients in the future.

The choice of methodology, whether it be qualitative or quantitative in nature, is entirely dependent on what the research question is. In some cases, a mixture of qualitative and quantitative methods can be used and this mixed methodology is becoming more popular in health-care research to provide a much wider view of the study concept so that it is more holistic.

Pros and cons of qualitative and quantitative methods

There have been, and still are, many arguments about the merits of the different methodologies in research. I would say that this is irrel-evant and that the most important factor to consider is that the most appropriate methodology is used to establish good-quality and valid results of the research question under study.

There are similarities between both methodologies. Some would argue that quantitative research is very limiting and only focuses on a very small area of the whole, but this is sometimes necessary. This is in comparison to qualitative studies, which are more holistic. This may be appropriate, depending on the research area and question that is trying to be answered by the study. There are many pros and cons of both methods in terms of data analysis. Some consider that the infor-mation gained from qualitative research is open to misinterpretation and bias from the researcher, while others consider that numerical data is good but wonder how this can be related to people's thoughts and feelings of a certain disease. The debate continues.

Conclusion

No matter what methodology is used, the overriding principle is *quality* and the protection of participants from any harm, be that physical or psychological. Any research that involves human subjects, such as the majority of healthcare research, needs ethical approval to ensure this.

Recap and recall

- Research is a process where new knowledge is discovered or facts confirmed
- Research is a process that involves a number of steps, including formation of the research question, searching the literature to see what has been done before, deciding on the methodology and which tools to use, finding your participants, doing a pilot study, adjusting your methods because of findings from the pilot study, collecting data, analysing data and discussing the findings and drawing conclusions from the results
- Two broad methods of research are used – qualitative and quantitative
- Qualitative research aims to gather information to enable the understanding of human behaviour. The data generated from such research are descriptive and are analysed to show themes that emerge
- There are a number of methodologies used in qualitative research and these include grounded theory, phenomenology, ethnography and action research
- Quantitative research aims to provide occurrences and facts. The data generated are numerical and are analysed using statistical and mathematical methods

- There are a number of methodologies used in quantitative research and these include clinical trials, cross-sectional studies, cohort studies and case studies

- What determines the methodology to be used in the research study is the research question, what the area of study is and what is to be investigated. Is it people's thoughts and feelings, or is it cause and effect, where numbers are required to prove the cause and effect?

Key terms

Bias The influence of factors other than those being studied. If the bias is not eliminated or minimised as much as possible, then the results of the study could be deemed invalid.

Cohort studies A method of research in which groups of people with a certain diagnosis and/or who are receiving a particular treatment are followed over time and compared with another group who do not have the diagnosis or are not receiving the treatment.

Control group This is a group of study participants who are recruited to the study to be compared with the experimental group, who undergo the intervention. The control group may be given a placebo, such as in drug trials.

Hawthorne effect This is a phenomenon that has been observed in research to occur when the participants are fully aware of being studied, observed or when they are asked a set of questions that might have some sort of consequences for them. This can affect the validity of the study.

Informed consent This is the process of ensuring that everyone participating in a research study is fully aware of what is going to happen. Participants are usually given the information verbally and also in a written format. They also understand that they can withdraw from involvement in the study at any time. This process usually requires a formal signature from the participant and also from the researcher to say that the information has been given.

Placebo This is a non-active substance or form of intervention used for the control group so that they can be compared to the experimental group.

Questionnaire This is a data collection tool that can be paper- or web-based. Respondents are asked to complete a series of structured question or items. Answers can be tick box format or open-ended questions depending on what type of information is required. The data can be numerical or narrative and descriptive depending on the design of the questionnaire.

Validity This is the extent to which the data, and its interpretation, reflects the phenomenon under investigation without any bias.

Post-test

You might like to test your knowledge and understanding with these questions. You will find the correct answers at the end of the book.

1. Name the stages in a typical research process.

2. Name three differences between qualitative and quantitative research.

3. Name three methodologies used in qualitative research.

4. Name three methodologies used in quantitative research.

5. What sort of data does qualitative research generate?

6. What sort of data does quantitative research generate?

References and further reading

Bowling, A. (2002) *Research Methods in Health; Investigating Health and Health Services*, 2nd edn. Berkshire: Open University Press.

Cormack, D., Gerrish, K., Lacey, A. (eds) (2006) *The Research Process in Nursing*, 5th edn. London: Blackwell Publishing.

Department of Health. (2001) *Research Governance Framework for Health and Social Care.* London: HMSO.

Doll, R., Peto, R., Boreham, J., Sutherland, I. (2004) Mortality in relation to smoking: 50 years' observations on male British doctors. *British Medical Journal,* **328**: 1519.

Glaser, B.G., Straus, A.L. (1999) *Discovery of Grounded Theory; Strategies for Qualitative Research.* London: Aldine Transaction.

Hek, G. (1994) The research process. *Journal of Community Nursing,* **8**(6): 4-6.

Kirk, K. (1996) Embarking on the research process; a guide. *Health Visitor,* **69**(9): 370-2.

Mays. N., Pope, C. (2000) Assessing quality in qualitative research. *British Medical Journal,* **320**: 50-2.

Meadows, K.A. (2003) So you want to do research? 1. An overview of the research process. *British Journal of Community Nursing,* **8**(8): 369-75.

Chapter 2

What is evidence and evidence-based practice?

AIMS

When you have read this chapter, you should understand:

- What evidence is
- Where evidence comes from
- How we find the evidence and what we do with it
- What needs to be considered when implementing the evidence into our clinical practice
- What is meant by the hierarchy of evidence

What is evidence?

Evidence is more than the findings from formal research projects. Rycroft-Malone *et al.* (2004) suggest that there are four distinct sources of evidence: one is research and the other three are clinical or professional experience, patients and their carers, and the local context in which you practise. This includes things such as audit and evaluation data, local professional networks and feedback from quality assurance programmes.

As healthcare professionals we need to draw upon all of these resources to ensure effective use of evidence in our work. We also need to know where to find it and what to do with it once we have found it. We also need to know how to apply the evidence, and where experience and judgement are central to this.

ACTIVITY 2.1

Are you aware of any audits or quality assurance programmes that have been carried out in your area of work?

Do you know who carried them out and why, and, more importantly, what the results were and the implications for practice?

If not, take some time to find this sort of information out and discover where such information is available in your organisation.

What is evidence-based practice?

We have clarified what we mean by evidence, but another commonly used term in today's health service is evidence-based practice. Other terms you may have heard are evidence-based care, evidence-based medicine and evidence-based nursing. Essentially they are the same, just terminology being applied to the different professions. The fundamental principle is that, as health professionals, we try and use the best evidence for the effective care of individuals, using it with the person's best interests in mind, to the best of our ability and in such a way that it is clear to others that we are doing it.

There are many definitions of evidence-based care, the first of which is a widely accepted definition by Sackett *et al.* (1996), defining evidence-based medicine as:

the conscientious, explicit and judicious use of current best practice in making decisions about the care of individual patients. The practice of evidence based medicine means integrating individual clinical expertise with the best available external clinical evidence from systematic research.   (Sackett *et al.*, 1996: p. 71)

This definition highlights the need to draw on both the professional's clinical experience and knowledge and the best external evidence, as neither is enough on its own. Clinical practice will become out of date if new evidence is not drawn upon. However, the clinician must be aware of what evidence is appropriate to their practice and this is an issue discussed later in this chapter. This definition does, however, provide some discussion and debate about the fact that although systematic research is considered the best-quality research (see section on 'The hierarchy of evidence', p. 24), it is not always available, especially in some areas of healthcare research such as health psychology and mental health nursing. It should also be ensured that patients are involved in decisions about their care.

An alternative definition provided by Muir Gray is:

an approach to decision making in which the clinician uses the best evidence available, in consultation with the patient, to decide upon the option which suits the patient best.   (Muir Gray, 1997)

In the current age of **clinical governance**, healthcare staff must strive to provide the best quality of care. There are many reasons why healthcare professionals need to engage with evidence-based practice and these include:

- The increasingly complex nature of healthcare decisions
- The Department of Health's directive that services and treatments should be based on the best evidence of what does and does not work (Department of Health, 1997)
- Compliance with codes of professional conduct
- The healthcare professional's ability to make informed judgements is of importance to patients to assist healthcare professionals in being valued members of the multidisciplinary team.

It is important that the evidence used is the most up to date and relevant. Research findings may not always be the best source of evidence in some cases, as there are some areas where research has not been carried out. There may be instances where research has been done, but the data are not relevant for your situation; for example, there may have been lots of research done to show that antibiotic A is the best for an ear infection. Unfortunately, your patient is allergic to antibiotic A. The GP decides to try antibiotic B, which he has found to work quite well from his experience, but it does not have the same research backing as antibiotic A. In this situation it is the next best option and is based on evidence from personal experience and from discussions with other healthcare professionals such as the pharmacist.

The overload of evidence – how do we deal with it?

It will not matter where you work in the health service, be it as a student nurse or as a consultant, a pharmacist or a manager, you will suffer the same snowstorm and overload of information from many different sources. The information, when it comes, is usually on a relevant topic (for example, guidelines on breast screening or information on the management of coronary heart disease) and is important, but the problem is that it has to be placed in the context of your own clinical area. Sometimes we need to be selective over what we read and apply a 'need to know' principle, owing to the enormous amount of information and the time pressures we have upon us. It is an impossible task to read every article that is published on a certain topic.

To practise evidence-based care we need to be critical and ask questions about the care we are providing and not just take for granted that it is the best way of doing it. We need to discover the reason that things are done in this way and see if the evidence supporting this is valid. So, when we have this overload of evidence, we need to have a systematic approach to dealing with it and a way of searching through it.

How do we search the evidence?

Evidence-based practice can be broken down into five stages.

1. *The question*: this is the recognition that there is a need for new information, and this information need has to be converted into an answerable question.

2. *Finding the evidence*: this is about searching for the right evidence and there are many databases that can be used to search the evidence. These include **CINAHL**, MEDLINE, Embase or databases within the **Cochrane library**. The skill lies in which terms or phrases you input into these databases for information. There is much advice available for you to do this, and any academic library in a university or college will have help and advice at hand. There are summaries available of best evidence and one good example of this is 'Clinical Evidence', which summarises the evidence for a broad range of conditions. Also, organisations such as **NICE** and **SIGN** produce guidelines with the evidence listed that was used to form them. *The Journal of Evidence Based Nursing* is another example and provides abstracts on the clinical application of research studies. The internet today aids in the efficiency of searching the literature, but you need to be aware of the process that you need to follow, and the librarian at your local hospital trust or college will assist you with this and provide guidance – a good place to start.

3. *Appraisal*: this is where the evidence you have gathered is **critically appraised** to determine its validity and potential usefulness. The fact that an article or research study has been published does not necessarily mean that it is valid or reliable, or even applicable to your clinical practice. Once you have found the evidence that will hopefully answer your question, the next stage is to critically appraise it to determine whether it is valid. Does the research answer the question it set out to answer, and does it provide answers to the question that *you* set out to answer? When appraising the evidence, the main questions to ask about the evidence/research are:

  a. Can the evidence or results of the research study be trusted? By this I mean have they been formed through an appropriate methodology during the research process?

  b. What is the evidence telling you and what does it mean?

  c. Does the research/evidence answer your question?

  d. Is it all relevant to your clinical practice?

There are many tools that have been developed to help you critically appraise research and evidence, whether qualitative or quantitative methodologies have been used. These include the CASP tools, which can be found at www.phru.nhs.uk/Pages/PHD/resources.htm and tools designed by the University of Salford, which can be found at www.fhsc.salford.ac.uk/hcprdu/critical-appraisal.htm.

4. *Acting on evidence*: this is where you have decided, following your critical appraisal, that the evidence is of good quality, and you will decide whether it should be incorporated into your clinical practice.

To help to incorporate this evidence into your clinical practice, you will need to draw upon your own expertise, experience and knowledge of your patient population and clinical area. You need to consider both the benefits and risks of implementing any changes, as well as the benefits and risks of excluding any alternatives. This decision cannot be made on your own. You need to work collaboratively with your patients, in consultation with the rest of the team and your manager. Change can be difficult to achieve if not approached in an appropriate way, and resistance to change can be a big problem. To minimise this you need to involve everyone concerned from the start, to ensure that change is made and sustained.

5. *Evaluation and reflection*: this is necessary to determine whether the action you have taken has achieved the desired results, and this is a fundamental part of healthcare practice.

Reflection and reflective practice are now terms which are well established in healthcare practice. Practitioners are encouraged and expected to reflect upon their role and their encounters with patients, their carers and other members of the healthcare team, to enhance their development. In terms of evidence-based practice, key areas to reflect upon are:

a. that you are asking an appropriate question; that the question you were requiring an answer to was indeed answerable and explicit enough to enable evidence to be collected;
b. that, in terms of finding the evidence, you searched the most appropriate resources and sites available and how easy or difficult the evidence was to find;
c. when it came to appraising and interpreting the evidence, that an appropriate tool was used and that your skills were adequate to enable an effective appraisal of the evidence and literature to be carried out, or is this an area where you need help and development of your own skills;
d. when you had appraised the evidence and came to act upon it in terms of your clinical practice, that you involved others, both within the healthcare team and also the patients and carers, and that the organisation and management was effective. If not, what could have been done differently? If it was implemented, what were the benefits and how are you going to ensure that this changed practice is sustained?

It must be remembered that evidence-based practice is all about questioning what you are doing. It is a continuous process which not only ensures the provision of best-quality care to patients, but also develops you as a healthcare professional, both personally and professionally.

Evidence-based practice is a continual process – once you have worked through one question, more questions develop that need to be answered. The diagram below illustrates this process.

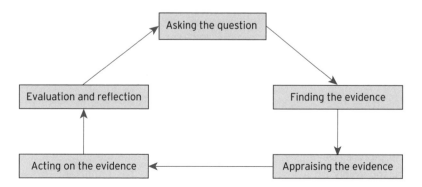

The hierarchy of evidence

One final area to mention is the hierarchy of evidence. This considers the best quality of evidence. This is graded in a hierarchy and the level of quality needs to be considered when doing a literature search or searching the evidence base. As discussed right at the start of this chapter, evidence comes in many forms and varies in quality. The hierarchy generally accepted is shown in the table below.

Rank	Methodology	Example/description
1	Systematic reviews and **meta-analyses**	These are review bodies of data, usually from randomised controlled trials, about a subject area. They use specific methodologies and employ statistical methods in their analysis
2	**Randomised controlled trials** (RCTs)	Clinical trials, which have a clear methodology, the use of randomisation of study participants and interventions and the use of control groups. They are usually published in **peer-reviewed journals**
3	**Case-controlled studies** and cross-sectional surveys	These are clinical trials without the randomisation used in RCTs. They will be published in peer-reviewed journals
4	**Non-experimental** designs, qualitative **studies**, e.g. cross-sectional surveys and case studies/reports	Non-numerical data are usually elicited from these studies (qualitative studies). They will be published in peer-reviewed journals. Although ranked fourth, they are important sources of evidence and, depending on the research area, are the only sources of data when quantitative studies are not able to be performed
5	Expert opinion	This includes opinions from well-respected authorities, based on clinical evidence, descriptive studies or reports from committees. They can include NICE guidelines, evidence-based local procedures and care pathways
6	Views of colleagues or peers	These views come from personal experience, observation and reflection on clinical practice

This is not to say that evidence at level 6 is useless. Many of the large RCTs are formed from personal observations made during clinical practice, and evidence from all levels plays a part in the overall picture. Obviously, however, you would not change your practice based solely on evidence from level 6. Finally, it is important to say that this hierarchy is not fixed in stone. It is only a generally recognised and accepted hierarchy. There is some debate over the relative positions of **systematic reviews** and large RCTs. In some people's eyes, RCTs are regarded as the most objective method of removing bias and producing comparable groups (as discussed in Chapter 1 on qualitative and quantitative research methodologies).

Conclusion

With the ever-increasing use of technology, the access to evidence is becoming easier and easier, as long as the healthcare professional has the skills and knowledge on how to search this evidence and evaluate it once they have retrieved it. All healthcare professionals have a professional duty to keep themselves updated and also to share evidence in the multidisciplinary team in which they work, to enable enhancement and continuation of evidence-based practice and the positive outcomes this should have on patient care and the efficient running of our health service.

Recap and recall

- There are four distinct sources of evidence in healthcare, these being from research, from clinical or professional experience, from patients and their carers and from the local context in which you practise, such as internal audits, local professional networks and feedback from quality assurance programmes

- As healthcare professionals we need to draw on all these sources of evidence. We also need to know where to find the evidence and what to do with it once we have found it and then how to apply it to our own practice

- Evidence-based practice is all about using the best evidence for the effective care of individuals, using it with the person's best

25

interests in mind, to the best of our ability and in such a way that it is clear to others that we are doing it

- In the current climate of clinical governance, healthcare staff must strive to provide the best-quality care that they can, drawing upon the available evidence

- Healthcare professionals need to engage with evidence-based practice owing to the increasing complexity of healthcare, because the Department of Health are dictating that care and services should be based on the best evidence, because we need to comply with codes of conduct and because we need to make informed judgements about the care we give and be part of an effective multidisciplinary care team

- Evidence-based practice does not mean that evidence is used only to change practice – it is also there to support existing practice and guard it against change

- Evidence-based practice can be broken down into five stages: (1) the question; (2) finding the evidence; (3) appraising the evidence; (4) acting on the evidence; and (5) evaluating the process and reflecting upon it. It is a continual process

- A hierarchy of evidence exists, which ranks the types of evidence in terms of quality. This is not set in stone and there is lots of debate about the ranking of some forms of evidence, such as qualitative evidence. It must be remembered that some areas of research cannot use quantitative methods because of their aims and their intended outcomes. A clinical decision should not only be based on the highest ranking forms of evidence but should pull from all sources and ranks.

Key terms

Case-controlled studies This method of research involves the comparison of a case (or person with a certain condition) and a person without the condition, but all other characteristics are similar (pair-matched control).

CINAHL This is a database of references to journals and papers dating back to 1982. The subject coverage focuses on nursing and midwifery journals but also includes primary journals for allied health professionals, such as physiotherapy, health education and nutrition.

Clinical governance This is a concept in the NHS designed to introduce a systematic approach to the delivery of high-quality healthcare.

Cochrane library An online database of high-quality evidence to inform healthcare decision-making. Includes evidence from meta-analyses and systematic reviews. These are recognised as the gold standard in evidence-based healthcare.

Critical appraisal A careful and thorough appraisal and review of strengths and weaknesses of a piece of research.

Meta-analysis A statistical technique for combining the findings of two or more clinical trials. It is used to assess the effectiveness of healthcare interventions.

NICE National Institute for Health and Clinical Excellence: this is part of the NHS. Its role is to provide patients, healthcare staff and the public with authoritative, robust and reliable guidance on current best practice.

Non-experimental studies Research in which data is collected without introducing any treatments or changes, i.e. the participants are being observed or are asked questions.

Peer-reviewed journals These journals are viewed as more authoritative and of higher academic quality than journals that have not been peer-reviewed. The journal articles have been reviewed by experts within the field prior to publication.

Randomised controlled trial (RCT) A form of experimental design where the study participants are randomly allocated into two groups, the experimental group and the control group. The experimental group receives the intervention or treatment that is being tested, whilst the control group receives an alternative or placebo. The outcomes of the two groups are compared and analysed using statistical methods to see the effect of the intervention.

SIGN Scottish Intercollegiate Guidelines Network. Develops evidence in the same way as NICE, for the NHS in Scotland.

Systematic review A method of summarising research evidence. All published and unpublished studies in a particular area are assessed for their scientific rigour and the findings are summarised in an unbiased and balanced manner.

Post-test

You might like to test your knowledge and understanding with these questions. You will find the correct answers at the end of the book.

1. What is evidence? What are some of the sources of evidence?

2. Define evidence-based practice.

3. What are the five stages of evidence-based practice?

4. Name two useful online databases that can be used to search the evidence.

5. What do you need to reflect upon in terms of evidence-based practice?

6. What is ranked first in the hierarchy of evidence?

7. What is ranked last in the hierarchy of evidence?

References and further reading

Department of Health. (1997) *The New NHS; Modern, Dependable.* London: HMSO.

Department of Health. (1998) *A First Class Service.* London: HMSO.

Department of Health. (2000) *Towards a Strategy for Nursing Research and Development: Proposals for Action.* London: HMSO.

Department of Health. (2006) *Best Research for Best Health: a New National Research Health Strategy.* London: HMSO.

Gerrish, K., Clayton, J. (2004) Promoting evidence-based practice; an organizational approach. *Journal of Nursing Management,* **12**: 114-23.

Greenhalgh, T. (2000) *How to Read a Paper: the Basics of Evidence Based Medicine*. London: BMJ Books.

Hendry, C., Farley, A. (1998) Reviewing the literature; a guide for students. *Nursing Standard*, **12**(44): 46-8.

McKibbon, K.A., Marks, S. (1998) Searching for the best evidence; part 1: where to look. *Evidence Based Nursing*, **1**(3): 68-9.

McKibbon, K.A., Marks, S. (1998) Searching for the best evidence; part 2: searching CINAHL and Medline. *Evidence Based Nursing*, **1**(4): 105-7.

Muir Gray, J.A. (1997) *Evidence-Based Healthcare: How to Make Health Policy and Management Decisions*. London: Churchill Livingstone.

Rycroft-Malone, J., Harvey, J.G., Seers, K. (2004) An explanation of the factors that influence the implementation of evidence into practice. *Journal of Clinical Nursing*, **13**(8): 913-24.

Sackett, D.L., Rosenberg, W.M.C., Gray, J.A.M., Richardson, W.S. (1996) Evidence based medicine; what it is and it isn't. *British Medical Journal*, **312**: 71-2.

Thompson, C. (2003) Clinical experience as evidence in evidence-based practice. *Journal of Advanced Nursing*, **43**(3): 230-7.

Websites

Department of Health Clinical Governance site
www.doh.gov.uk/clinicalgovernance

Clinical evidence
www.clinicalevidence.com/ceweb/about/index.jsp6Feb2006

National Library for Health (NLH)
www.library.nhs.uk

Centre for evidence-based nursing
www.york.ac.uk/healthsciences/centres/evidence/cebn.htm

Cochrane collaboration
www.cochrane.org/index0.htm

National Institute for Health and Clinical Excellence (NICE)
www.nice.org.uk

Critical Appraisal Skills Programme (CASP)
www.phru.nhs.uk/Pages/PHD/resources.htm

Centre for evidence-based medicine
www.cebm.net/index.aspx?o=1157

University of Salford, critical appraisal tools
http://fhsc.salford.ac.uk/hcprdu/critical-appraisal.htm

Chapter 3

Why do we need an evidence base in our clinical practice?

AIMS

When you have read this chapter, you should understand:

- The importance of quality patient care
- The professional responsibility involved in quality patient care
- The principles of clinical governance and continued professional development
- Change management and the drivers for change in the health service
- Public involvement in any change in healthcare services and implementation of evidence base into clinical practice

What is quality care?

There are a few terms bandied around that relate to quality care – one is **clinical effectiveness**. The Department of Health (1996) defines clinical effectiveness as the extent to which specific clinical interventions, when deployed in the field for a particular patient or population, do what they are intended to do; that is, to maintain or improve health and secure the greatest possible health gain from the resources available.

But what does this mean in terms of our everyday clinical practice? It relates to the decisions we make about the care we give to individual patients, how we run our services and plan the services that we deliver. We need to ensure that they are all driven by evidence to guarantee they are effective, enabling all clinical practitioners to achieve positive and beneficial outcomes to all, not just the patient and the carers but to the staff, the managers and also the cost and resources.

Clinical effectiveness is all about achieving improved outcomes of care. Without evidence how would we achieve this? However, new evidence alone cannot guarantee clinical effectiveness and there are many other factors involved, which are illustrated in Figure 3.1.

Many of these factors are interlinked and cannot exist or develop without the other, and many, such as policies and guidelines development and professional issues, are developed more effectively with the increased academic capabilities of nurses and other healthcare professionals.

Although in the past the focus of healthcare professionals was on achieving financial goals, this is an important factor in the equation, but now more attention is paid to achieving increased **quality** of care. The increased access to the internet and intense media interest mean that the public have much greater access to information on the effectiveness of treatments and can challenge clinicians on treatment decisions. On the other hand, this can also enable people to take more responsibility for their own health and take on self-care through informed choice.

Patients and the public also have greater involvement in the planning and evaluation of health services, as do the universities that provide the training for healthcare professionals. User involvement is an area that universities are now assessed on by professional bodies, such as the Nursing and Midwifery Council, as is the develop-

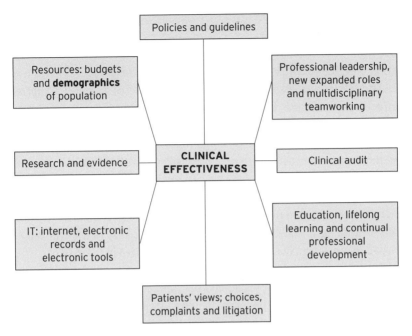

Figure 3.1 Factors involved in achieving clinical effectiveness.

ment of courses for the purpose of training and educating healthcare professionals.

In amongst all this we must never forget about the economic and financial implications of quality evidence-based care. The NHS, like other publicly funded services, is cost-limited. Various changes in the overall population structure, advances in the sophistication of treatments available and the increased expectations of the public have all contributed to escalating demand for service. Therefore we need to be acutely aware of the need to do more with less.

ACTIVITY 3.1

Quality of care – think of a situation when you have done something and wondered why you have done it that way and what was the evidence for this?

....

....

....

The Department of Health (1998b), published *Achieving Effective Practice*, which identified a wide range of benefits to patients, nurses and the NHS from increased clinical effectiveness. It is thus true to say that clinical effectiveness is an integral part of care delivery.

There is a particularly cruel irony in the rise of hospital-acquired infections in an era in which evidence-based practice is generally accepted as a key component of modern healthcare; evidence-based approaches to preventing cross-infection were already clearly evident in the nineteenth century. For example, in the 1840s Semmelweis's insistence that doctors performing autopsies should wash their hands before going to deliver babies was associated with a dramatic reduction in mortality due to sepsis, from over 20% to 3%. Similarly, it was observation that led John Snow in the 1840s to pinpoint a water tap in Broad Street as a cause of the outbreak of cholera in London.

These two examples from the nineteenth century encapsulate the variety of domains of professional health practice that can and should be evidence-based, but they also demonstrate how powerful **reflective questioning** and acutely observant practitioners can uncover evidence with their own everyday practice, which, when acted upon, can improve health.

ACTIVITY 3.2

Think of any situations that you may have come across like this.

....

....

....

....

What are the drivers for evidence-based practice and quality care?

There are a number of drivers for pushing forward the issues related to quality care and clinical effectiveness. These can all be analysed

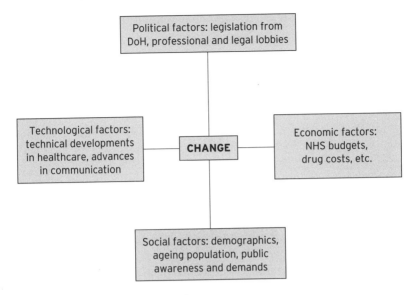

Figure 3.2   The PEST framework.

and evaluated by using a tool such as PEST, which stands for political, economic, social and technological, these being the factors/areas we need to consider when considering any analysis and change. This is illustrated in Figure 3.2.

Changing practice requires energy, motivation and support from others, which need to be sustainable over time. There are many drivers for change, as illustrated in Figure 3.2, but encapsulating all of these and managing the conflicts that may arise is challenging.

When managing a change in practice, there are several key considerations, the first being patient benefit, which is an intrinsic feature of the process of implementing evidence base into practice. Secondly, changes need to be congruent with the objectives of the organisation and accepted as a current priority that warrants the level of expenditure of time and other resources.

ACTIVITY 3.3

Have you ever been in a position to witness a change in practice or a change in the way things are done? Did it run smoothly? If so, what helped this; if not, what could have been done better and what were the barriers? Were all the factors of the PEST framework considered?

....

....

....

....

....

Clinical governance – what is it?

Because of the continued increased pressure upon resources and the need to ensure that services offered are appropriate in meeting needs and demands, the government has pushed for the delivery of clinically effective care. In 1997 the Department of Health published *The New NHS: Modern and Dependable*, which started a shift of focus onto the quality of care, so that excellence could be guaranteed to all patients.

There was an emphasis on the area of clinical effectiveness as part of the overall strategy of clinical governance. *A First Class Service: Quality in the New NHS* (Department of Health, 1998a) developed these concepts and clinical governance was described as: '. . . a framework through which NHS organisations are accountable for continuously improving the quality of their services and safeguarding high standards of care by creating an environment in which excellence in clinical care can flourish (Department of Health, 1998a: p. 6).

The Royal College of Nursing (RCN) have also highlighted three key dimensions of clinical governance:

1. Improved quality

2. Management of risk and performance

3. Systems of accountability and responsibility.

They concluded by saying that clinical governance was everyone's business.

ACTIVITY 3.4

Have you seen evidence of these three key dimensions? If so, in what circumstances? For example, was there a clinical incident where a clinical risk assessment was carried out? If you are not sure, find out, as these are three important areas to be aware of in your work environment and your professional role.

....

....

....

....

....

The National Institute for Health and Clinical Excellence (NICE) was launched because it was felt that there was a need for clear standards for clinical services. NICE was launched to review evidence and to issue national guidance in relation to specific treatments or investigations, based on evidence of clinical and cost-effectiveness. The development of the **National Service Frameworks** (NSFs) was also initiated to provide clear standards and guidance for care relating to specific conditions or patient groups, e.g. coronary heart disease and diabetes.

ACTIVITY 3.5

What NSFs are used in your clinical area of work? If there aren't any find out why. Maybe there isn't one written or maybe there is one but it hasn't been used for some reason.

....

....

....

....

....

37

It is expected that key components of clinical governance will be developed by the health service. These include:

1. Clinical **audit**
2. Clinical effectiveness
3. Risk management
4. Research and development
5. Education, training and continuing professional development (CPD)
6. Staffing and staff management
7. Openness and patient involvement.

ACTIVITY 3.6

Look at how these have been developed in the area in which you work or have worked. Ask about how these activities are carried out, i.e. is there a PALS (Patient Advice and Liaison Services) in your trust? What facilities are there for CPD of staff? How are clinical audits carried out and what is done with the information generated from these?

....

....

....

....

....

....

Another area that has been developed since the introduction of clinical governance is clinical guidelines, protocols and care pathways. They play a key role in clinical effectiveness and are based on evidence generated in the specific area of interest from the protocol or guideline. The pros and cons of these will be addressed in Chapter 4 in more detail.

What do the public think of quality care?

There have been some very well documented media portrayals of downfalls in the quality of care provided, and this has been highlighted in the increase in litigation to the health service. You need to justify the care that you give and this will protect you and your employer from litigation. There is a National Health Service Litigation Authority (NHSLA) which deals with such claims and the NHS Redress Bill (2005) states that patient/clients who suffer as a result of NHS mistakes could receive up to £20,000 compensation without going to court. This really illustrates the importance of quality care and the use of evidence base in the care we give.

To make a successful claim for negligence against a health and social care provider, the patient has to demonstrate that the health-care provider failed in their duty of care and that this failure led to harm. The courts have consistently ruled that such a failure occurs if the health and social care provider has not provided care that is evidence-based (Dimond, 2009). Therefore, if you are able to provide a good rationale or explanation for your practice, and show that it is an essential component of the concept of evidence-based practice, you will prevent yourself from becoming involved in any legal proceedings.

Increasingly, the public demands more and more information about the various services available to them. There is a demand for greater respect for openness and accountability to patients and the public. There needs to be comprehensive easily understood information, spelling out both advantages and disadvantages, so that informed decisions can be made.

The Department of Health has also written guidance on consent, which should always be followed (Department of Health, 2001). Both *The Patient's Charter* (Department of Health, 1991) and the new NHS complaints system (Department of Health, 1996, 2004) provide the impetus for the need for the clinical effectiveness of interventions to be a standard expectation for patients and the public. This was also emphasised in the Commission for Health Improvement clinical governance inspections, and subsequent policy documents (Department of Health, 2003, 2004) have supported further development of patient and public involvement in the work of NICE. Most organisations and trusts now house some form of patient or public involvement in clinical governance processes; for example, through patient or public representation on committees or through patient forums or PALS.

Education and training and healthcare professionals and Continuing Professional Development (CPD)

With the move from the old schools of nursing into higher education, and now with the move to an all degree profession, the view of nursing as a profession has been changed in a positive way. Because of these moves in educational standards of the nursing profession, there is more recognition of research and academic scholarship to support clinically effective care.

Nurses are given opportunities for development and are encouraged to be more analytical. They have developed skills of critical enquiry and are taught about evidence-based practice during their preregistration training, so that these principles are embedded during their development into trained members of staff.

Increasing numbers of nurses are also pursuing continuing educational achievements, with postregistration education and training, which has the support of the Department of Health from the document on postregistration nursing education (Department of Health, 2008).

Nurses are also taking on expanded roles such as physical assessment and prescribing, which were previously purely medical roles. With this links their continual education and updating, and knowledge and responsibility for the roles undertaken.

Education and learning, however, is not a single process but a continual one. New developments are always present in the health service, new services are being developed or changed, and guidelines developed and implemented for better patient outcomes. All these developments are based on the ever-present availability of new evidence. Health professionals, therefore, need to update and refresh their knowledge and skills continually.

The Department of Health and the Nursing and Midwifery Council have published documents on CPD and lifelong learning and we have a professional responsibility to ensure our continued professional development.

ACTIVITY 3.7

What education updates and training have you done in the past 12 months? Do you feel that there are areas that you could do with more knowledge about? Do you know how to and who to approach for this education and the practicalities of gaining funding and time to achieve this from your clinical area? If not, then find this out.

....

....

....

....

....

....

Conclusion

So let us now return to the question posed by the title of this chapter – why do we need evidence-based practice?

In this chapter we can see that it is the cornerstone of quality care, but we can also see that this brings about change in the health service, which needs to be managed effectively. We can see that evidence-based practice originated from the principles of clinical governance, which also links in with the initial and ongoing education of healthcare professionals, to develop the evidence at the same time as techno-logical advances in healthcare. We can also see now how education of staff into new expanded and advanced roles contributes to the con-tinual development of evidence and quality of care.

Finally, we must not forget the importance of public involvement in the development of evidence-based care. The modern philosophy of multidisciplinary teamworking, public involvement and feedback, and audit of healthcare provision continues to drive forward evidence-based practice and, ultimately, higher quality of care.

Recap and recall

- Clinical effectiveness is the extent to which specific clinical interventions, when deployed in the field of a particular patient, or population, do what they are intended to do. That is, they maintain or improve health and secure the greatest possible health gain from the resources available (Department of Health, 1996)

- Factors involved in achieving clinical effectiveness include resources, research and evidence, policies and guidelines, clinical audit, professionalism, education, IT and patients' views

- Economic and financial implications of quality evidence-based care must not be forgotten, as the NHS is publicly funded and is cash-limited

- The vision for nursing in the twenty-first century is for all nurses to seek out evidence and apply it in their everyday practice, with an increasing proportion actively participating in research and development, and some developing into research leaders (Department of Health, 2000, 2006)

- There are a number of drivers for pushing forward the issues related to quality care and clinical effectiveness. These can all be analysed and evaluated using a tool such as PEST

- Changing practice requires energy, motivation and support from others, which need to be sustainable over time

- Clinical governance is a framework through which NHS organisations are accountable for continuously improving the quality of their services and safeguarding high standards of care by creating an environment in which excellence in clinical care can flourish (Department of Health, 1998a)

- The Royal College of Nursing highlights three key dimensions of clinical governance: (1) improving quality; (2) management of risk and performance; (3) systems of accountability and responsibility

- NICE was launched by the government to review evidence and issue national guidance in relation to specific treatments or investigations, based on evidence of clinical cost-effectiveness

- The development of NSFs was also initiated to provide clear standards and guidance for care relating to specific conditions or patient groups, e.g. coronary heart disease, diabetes

- Key components of clinical governance include clinical audit, clinical effectiveness, risk management, research and development, education, training and continuing professional development, staffing and staff management, openness and patient involvement (Department of Health, 1998a)

- Both *The Patient's Charter* (Department of Health, 1991) and the new NHS Complaints System (Department of Health, 1996, 2004) provide the impetus for the need for the clinical effectiveness of interventions to be a standard expectation for patients and the public

- Most organisations and trusts have some form of patient or public involvement in clinical governance processes, e.g. through patient or public representation on committees or through patient forums or Patient Advice and Liaison Services (PALS)

- Health professionals need continually to update their knowledge and skills through evidence-based practice.

Key terms

Audit A way of reviewing a situation to check that all aspects are achieved. If it is highlighted that this is not the case, then measures can be taken to remedy the situation.

Clinical effectiveness About achieving improved outcomes of care and ensuring a quality service to patients and clients.

Demographics A description of the characteristics of a population such as age, gender, living accommodation, status of employment, etc.

National Service Frameworks Documents developed by NICE to provide clear standards and guidance for care relating to specific conditions or patient groups, e.g. diabetes.

Quality A degree or standard of excellence.

Reflective questioning Allows individuals to reflect aloud, to reflect on both positive and negative aspects of a situation and to gain feedback to expand and extend thinking through follow-up.

Post-test

You might like to check your knowledge and understanding with these questions. You will find the correct answers at the end of the book.

1. What is clinical effectiveness?

2. What is clinical governance?

3. What is the link between evidence-based practice and clinical governance?

4. Name four components of clinical governance.

5. Name a tool that can be used when implementing a change in an organisation. What factors need to be taken into account during this process?

6. Why is evidence important to quality care?

References and further reading

Department of Health. (1991) *The Patient's Charter*. London: HMSO.

Department of Health. (1996) *Promoting Clinical Effectiveness: a Framework for Action in and through the NHS*. Leeds: NHS Executive.

Department of Health. (1997) *The New NHS: Modern and Dependable*. London: HMSO.

Department of Health. (1998a) *A First Class Service: Quality in the New NHS*. London: HMSO.

Department of Health. (1998b) *Achieving Effective Practice: a Clinical Effectiveness and Research Information Pack for Nurses, Midwives and Health Visitors*. Leeds: NHS Executive.

Department of Health. (2000) *Towards a Strategy for Nursing Research and Development: Proposals for Action.* London: HMSO.

Department of Health. (2001) *Good Practice in Consent, Achieving the NHS Plan Committment to Patient Centred Practice.* HSC 2001/023. London: HMSO.

Department of Health. (2003) *The NHS Improvement Plan: Putting People at the Heart of Public Services.* London: HMSO.

Department of Health. (2004) *The NHS Complaints System.* London: HMSO.

Department of Health. (2005) *Redress Bill.* London: HMSO.

Department of Health. (2006) *Best Research for Best Health: a New National Research Health Strategy.* London: HMSO.

Department of Health. (2008) *Post Registration Nurse Education.* London: HMSO.

Department of Health./NHS Modernisation Agency. (2003) *The Essence of Care: Patient-focused Bench Marks for Clinical Governance.* London: HMSO.

Dimond, B. (2009) *Legal Aspects of Nursing,* 5th edn. Harlow: Pearson Education.

Gerrish, K., Clayton, J. (2004) Promoting evidence-based practice; an organizational approach. *Journal of Nursing Management,* **12**: 114–23.

Grol, R. (1997) Beliefs and evidence in changing clinical practice. *British Medical Journal,* **315**: 418–21.

NHS Executive. (1996) *Clinical Guidelines: Using Clinical Guidelines to Improve Patient Care Within the NHS.* Leeds: NHS Executive.

Pearson, M. (2000) Making a difference through research; how nurses can turn the vision into reality (editorial). *NT Research,* **5**(2): 85–6.

Plowman, R., Graves, N., Griffith, M. (1999) The socio-economic burden of hospital acquired infections occurring in patients admitted to selected specialities of a district general hospital in England and the national burden imposed. *Journal of Hospital Infection,* **47**(3): 198–209.

Rycroft-Malone, J., Harvey, G., Seers, K. (2004) An exploration of the factors that influence the implementation of evidence into practice. *Journal of Clinical Nursing,* **13**(8): 913–24.

Upton, T., Brooks, B. (1995) *Managing Change in the NHS.* London: Kogan Page.

Chapter 4

Clinical guidelines and the need for clinical audit

AIMS

When you have read this chapter, you should understand:

- What clinical guidelines are
- What the advantages and disadvantages of clinical guidelines are
- What clinical audit is
- How clinical audit relates to quality patient care
- How evidence links into the audit trail and clinical practice

What are clinical guidelines?

Clinical guidelines are '... systematically developed statements to assist practitioner decisions about appropriate health care for specific clinical circumstances' (Field and Lohr, 1990: p. 5).

Clinical guidelines can be written for specific conditions (for example, asthma, diabetes or angina), for symptoms such as pain or breathlessness and for procedures such as urinary catheterisation or arterial line insertion.

Guidelines can help to standardise care. For example, the British Asthma Guidelines, developed by the British Thoracic Society (BTS) and the Scottish Intercollegiate Guidelines Network (SIGN) (BTS/SIGN, 2010), reviewed the evidence base on all different aspects of asthma care and management and wrote guidelines which are seen as gold standard for the management of people with asthma all over the UK. Clinical guidelines such as these are based on the best evidence available. They are designed to help health professionals in their work, but they do not replace their knowledge, skills and clinical judgement.

ACTIVITY 4.1

Look at the guidelines you use in your clinical area and look at the evidence which was used to develop them.

....

....

....

....

The aims of clinical guidelines overall are to improve the quality of healthcare. They provide recommendations for the treatment and care of people by health professionals and they are used to develop standards to access the clinical practice of individual health professionals. They can also be used in the education and training of health professionals and to help patients make informed choices and decisions about their care, thus enhancing communication between the patient and the health professional.

Clinical guidelines can also help to defend clinicians in **litigation** suits. If a health professional treats a patient in accordance with an evidence-based guideline and the patient's condition deteriorates, then the healthcare professional can claim that he did not cause harm through neglect as he was working under evidence-based guidelines and there would be no case of litigation. If, on the other hand, the healthcare professional made clinical decisions outside the recommended guidance and if he did not have the evidence to back this up, then he would be held accountable for his actions.

Characteristics of clinical guidelines

The NHS Centre for Review and Dissemination (1994) recommend that if guidelines are to be effective then they should ensure that as many as possible of the following characteristics are met:

a. *Validity*: the evidence used to formulate the guideline is valid and appropriate

b. *Cost-effectiveness*: guidelines should include/take into account costs and not just look at benefits or resources, which could be impractical

c. *Reproducibility*: given the same evidence, another guideline group would produce similar recommendations

d. *Reliability*: given the same clinical circumstances, a clinician would apply the recommendations set out in the guideline in a similar way

e. *Representative development*: that the group that develops the guidelines includes representatives from a broad range involved in that area

f. *Clinical applicability*: the target population is defined in accordance with the evidence

g. *Clinical flexibility*: guidelines identify exceptions and indicate how patient preferences are to be incorporated into decision-making

h. *Clarity*: guidelines use precise definitions, unambiguous language and user-friendly formats

i. *Meticulous documentation*: guidelines record participants, assumptions and methods and link recommendations to the available evidence

j. *Scheduled review*: state when and how the guideline is to be reviewed

k. *Utilisation review*: indicate ways in which adherence to recommendations can be sensibly monitored.

It is obviously then a very intense task, when developing guidelines, to ensure that they meet these criteria. It can be very resource-intensive and timely. The stages of guideline development usually include:

1. Selection of guideline topic
2. Composition of the guideline development group
3. Defining the scope of the guideline
4. Systematic literature review
5. Formation of recommendations
6. Consultation and peer review
7. Presentation and dissemination
8. Local implementation
9. Audit and review.

Introducing the guideline

Once the guideline is ready for use, there are two stages that it has to go through to enable it to be introduced into practice: dissemination and implementation. Dissemination is where various methods are employed to make the guideline available to target users. This can be done by publication in journals and sending the guideline to targeted individuals and education events and workshops.

Implementation is a means of ensuring that users subsequently act upon the recommendations. When designing an implementation strategy it is necessary to be aware of barriers to behavioural change, which can include both structural and attitudinal factors. Audit and feedback can also affect the behaviour of those for whom the guidelines are appropriate.

What are the advantages and disadvantages of clinical guidelines?

This section will be divided into advantages and disadvantages for patients, healthcare professionals and healthcare systems.

So, what are the potential benefits and advantages of clinical guidelines? The overriding benefit of clinical guidelines is that they improve the quality of care that is received by patients and users of the health service. Whether we can definitely claim this to be true is not clear, as everyone involved in the use of clinical guidelines has their own perceptions on what quality care is. So we can only realistically talk about 'potential' and 'likely' advantages and benefits, which can be classified under the the following sections.

Potential benefits to the patients

The greatest benefit here is to improved health outcomes and outcomes to the care and service delivery that patients receive from the health service and its personnel. Clinical guidelines are evidence-based and, through the evaluation of the best available evidence interventions, treatments and processes of care that have been proved to be effective are highlighted while ineffective ones are discouraged. Through this there should be a reduction in **rates of mortality** and **morbidity** and increased quality of life for patients and users of the health service.

Guidelines can also improve the consistency of care, as it has been shown that patients with identical clinical conditions are treated differently depending on their geographical location, the hospital or clinic visited and the health professional seen. This has a negative impact, not only on the trust and confidence of patients, but can lead to serious errors occurring.

Some clinical guidelines have leaflets, audiotapes and videos attached, which are available in different languages. They are also published in condensed versions in laymen's terms in the form of articles in magazines and newspapers and on the internet. There is an increased drive to develop public awareness of what to expect in terms of healthcare. This can empower patients to make more informed healthcare choices and to consider their personal needs and preferences in selecting the best options.

Clinical guidelines can also draw attention to under-recognised health problems, clinical services and preventative interventions and to neglected patient populations and high risk groups. By doing this, it can prompt the treating of conditions, and new roles for healthcare professionals may be developed. Clinical guidelines developed with attention to the public good can promote distributive justice, advocating better delivery of services to those in need. Also, in a cash-limited healthcare service, clinical guidelines that improve the efficiency of healthcare free up resources needed for other services and wastage is reduced.

Potential benefits to healthcare professionals

Clinical guidelines have an important role to play in helping with clinical decisions made by healthcare professionals. They do this because they offer recommendations for clinicians who may be uncertain about how to proceed, they overturn the beliefs of some accustomed to outdated practices, they improve the consistency of care and provide authoritative recommendations that reassure practitioners about the appropriateness of their treatment decisions and policies.

Evidence-based guidelines provide information to practitioners about the most beneficial interventions and treatment options, and also inform them of the quality of the evidence used to base these recommendations on, using the hierarchy of evidence format. Through this they also draw attention to wasteful and dangerous practices to safeguard patients.

Guidelines can also be used as an assessment tool in audit. Retrospective examination of clinical practice can act as an alert to the compliance with recommendations from the guidelines on best clinical practice and highlight dangerous divergences.

Researchers in healthcare welcome clinical guidelines because, through the evaluation of the evidence in the development of the guideline, gaps in evidence will be identified, leading to areas where research should be focused. The evaluation and review of the evidence will also highlight design and methodological faults in studies already published in an area, again identifying areas for further research to be carried out. It could be hard to identify these gaps in the evidence base if it were not for the development of clinical guidelines.

Finally, clinical guidelines can be used in a medicolegal situation for clinicians. If a patient comes to harm, clinicians' actions may be judged against recommendations given in evidence-based guidelines. If the clinician has followed such guidelines, then this could protect them from being sued for negligence. Obviously the opposite could be true if the clinician did not follow these recommendations.

Potential benefits for healthcare systems

Healthcare systems that provide services, and government bodies and private insurers that pay for them, may find that clinical guidelines may be effective in improving efficiency (often by standardising care) and optimising value for money. By introducing a clinical guideline and hence standardising care, the healthcare provider can save money on resources such as staff, drugs, surgery and other procedures and make the service provided more financially viable.

Public confidence and trust is a big issue in the health service. Therefore publicising to the public that a healthcare service follows evidence-based guidelines can help to enhance this confidence and trust, and relays messages of commitment to excellence and quality in the care and services provided.

Potential limitations and disadvantages of clinical guidelines

The most significant limitation and disadvantage from a clinical guideline is if the recommendations within it are wrong, or they may be wrong for that individual patient and the clinician has not realised it. This can happen because the guideline developers, reviewing all the evidence, may find that there is evidence lacking or it may be inconclusive. It may be misleading and therefore misinterpreted. This may be because of methodological and design flaws in the research study or from bias that may have been introduced into the research study from the researchers themselves or from the participants taking part in the study.

Guideline development groups may lack sufficient time and resources to scrutinise every piece of research in detail. They may also lack some of the skills. Their judgements may be subjective, especially when obvious deficits and possible harms are weighed against the benefits. We also need to consider that decisions about the recommendations made may be influenced by the developers' clinical experience and background, and this may also depend upon the composition and membership of the guideline development group.

We must also remember that the good of the patients may not be the only consideration in the recommendations given. Factors such as cost, societal needs and government policies may also drive the recommendations given in clinical guidelines.

Potential disadvantages to patients

The greatest danger to patients is if their care is guided by flawed guidelines, for obvious reasons. Guidelines can also sometimes be very inflexible and therefore the clinician using them cannot adapt them for individual patient needs. This is the case for 'blanket' recommendations, which can lead to inappropriate care if clinicians do not have the knowledge or expertise to interpret them to accommodate for individual circumstances. This highlights the importance of shared decision-making and working as a **multidisciplinary team** and also involving the patients in their care.

Lay versions of guidelines can be inappropriately worded and can confuse patients and their families. This can also harm the doctor-patient relationship when inappropriate demands are placed on the healthcare professional by the patient and their family from what they may have read or believe they have read.

Potential disadvantages to healthcare professionals

Flawed clinical guidelines compromise the quality of care that can be given by the healthcare professional. They may be forced to base their care on such guidelines and not diverge away, due to costs and available resources. Their clinical decisions can be affected, and time and money can be wasted on ineffective treatments. Sometimes clinicians can find guidelines inconvenient and untimely to use even if they are correct. There can also be conflicting advice in clinical guidelines on the same condition coming from different professional bodies – which advice do you follow then?

Some clinical guidelines can be seen as a tool acting against the healthcare professional and their clinical decisions. Auditors and managers may judge the quality of care given purely on the advice given by clinical guidelines. This is unfair and it should be stressed that guidelines only offer guidance and are not a strict set of rules to be followed. Clinicians' experiences should also be taken into the equation.

Guidelines that reduce a care pathway into a series of yes or no answers seriously damage the outcomes that patients may achieve and do not take into consideration the complexity of some medical conditions and, indeed, patients with multiple morbidities. Guidelines can sometimes state that certain treatments or diagnostic tests lack substantial evidence to back them. This can lead to funding bodies inappropriately withdrawing funding for a treatment which has given patients benefit for years.

Potential disadvantages for healthcare systems

Some guidelines are developed without consideration for costs, and therefore may recommend costly treatment options which are unaffordable to healthcare systems. Due consideration for costs always needs to be considered. If the lay public believe that they should have a certain treatment because it is recommended by a clinical guideline, the public uproar and fall in trust of the healthcare providers can be damaging. We are all aware of media coverage of such cases.

Overall, clinical guidelines can be effectively used to deliver positive patient care, as long as they are developed effectively and appropriately, taking all the considerations mentioned above into account. It must be remembered that, at the end of the day, clinical guidelines are only one option for improving quality of patient care.

What is clinical audit?

One definition of clinical audit is 'A quality improvement process that seeks to improve patient care and outcomes through systematic review of care against explicit criteria and the implementation of change' (NICE/CHI, 2002).

Clinical audit is an integral part of clinical governance, discussed in previous chapters, and is carried out by people involved in the treatment of patients. This does not have to be a nurse or a doctor. It is, in a nutshell, the measurement of practice against agreed standards and implementing change to ensure that all patients receive care to the same standard.

This all sounds very clear and simple, but there may be many challenges facing all concerned, especially if there are no clear criteria based on evidence on which to assess patient care against. This is where clinical guidelines can be used.

Medical audit was introduced in 1989 with the White Paper *Working for Patients* (Department of Health, 1989), which stated that systematic peer review of medical care should be part of the routine clinical practice for all doctors. This has obviously expanded now into a multidisciplinary approach. The clinical effectiveness agenda (Department of Health, 1996) was introduced in 1996 and it also highlighted the importance of evidence-based standards as a basis for all audit topics.

There is an abundance of terms bandied around, such as audit, research, service evaluation and service improvement. It can be very confusing to understand what they all mean and what the difference is between them. They are also sometimes misused, which adds to the confusion. To try and clarify this somewhat, the following are definitions for each of the terms.

Audit: aims to improve the quality of local patient care and clinical outcomes through review of practice against evidence-based standards, and the implementation of change where subsequently indicated. Questions asked in the audit process can be 'are we following best practice?' 'what is happening to the patients as a result?'

Research: aims to derive new knowledge which is potentially generalisable or transferable. A question to be asked in research is 'what is best practice?'

Service evaluation: aims to judge a service's effectiveness/efficiency through assessment of its aims, activities, outcomes and costs. It may also be called 'bench marking' or 'organisational audit'. A question to be asked in service evaluation could be 'has this service been a success?'

Service improvement: aims to improve patient care through continuous improvement of outcomes by focusing on quality and safety. It may also be referred to as 'service development'. A question that may be asked as part of service improvement is 'how can we make this service safer, more efficient and better for patients?'

In terms of the methodology used in each of these processes, audit addresses clearly defined audit questions using a robust methodology, usually asking whether a specific standard has been met. Results are very specific and local to where the audit has been carried out, which can be individual wards or units. Research addresses clearly defined questions and hypotheses using systematic and rigorous processes, as described in Chapter 1. It is designed so that it can be replicated and results can be generalised to other groups; for example, a trial may be held of a new drug on a group of patients with a specific disease. If it proves to be effective then it can be recommended to people with the same disease state.

Service evaluation addresses specific questions about the service concerned. Again, like audit, results are specific and local. Service improvement includes awareness and engagement of individuals and teams so there is agreement that improvement is necessary. Analysis of current systems, understanding current problems and capacity, agreeing steps to improve, developing a project implementation plan and ensuring changes are sustained are all part of the methodology of service improvement.

The end result is that audit generates evidence to demonstrate level of competence within agreed standards. This may lead to changes in practice. Research generates evidence to refute, support or develop a hypothesis, and may lead to development of new evidence and science which drives new practices. Service evaluation generates evidence of effectiveness of a service which may lead to service redesign and reconfiguration. Finally, service improvement generates evidence of improvements by comparing new service performance against a baseline, provides ideas for improvements and demonstrates skills transfer.

The audit cycle

Clinical audit is not a one-off exercise, but a continuous cycle of quality improvement. From one cycle of clinical audit a change in practice may be identified. An action plan is then put in place to achieve this desired change. This new change needs then to be monitored and reviewed again to ensure that it is achieving what it is expected to achieve.

The audit cycle can be represented as a cycle such as the one given below:

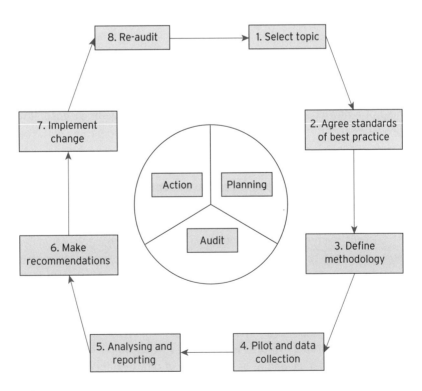

Hence, to be effective clinical audit requires:

1. Evidence-based standards
2. A multidisciplinary team approach
3. Monitoring of practice
4. Commitment to change.

None of the above four essential requirements can work on its own. They are all intertwined. The commitment to change is a major stepping stone and, without clinicians, administrators, managers, fund holders and patient groups all being involved as part of the change, it will not succeed. These groups of people cannot be passive and be outside the change process; they need to be involved from the start.

Also, without the evidence base to provide incentive for the change, it will not happen and this leads us back to the start of the book where we spoke about evidence, what it is and where it comes from. Without this basic understanding of evidence and evidence base, we cannot relate to any evidence-based care approaches that are used in our clinical practice.

ACTIVITY 4.2

Do you know who carries out the clinical audit in your area of work? If not, find out and find out what audit trails they have undertaken and how this will affect your day-to-day care.

....

....

....

....

....

Conclusion

After reading this chapter and undertaking the activities suggested, you can now begin to see how the evidence generated from research feeds back into clinical practice and patient care. There are differing opinions on clinical guidelines, but hopefully you will now have a broader understanding of the advantages and disadvantages of them. It all depends on the quality of the guideline produced. These statements cannot be applied as a broad blanket for all clinical guidelines. Read some clinical guidelines and see what you think. Now you can start to analyse them more and understand their development processes and quality in relation to clinical practice and patient care.

Finally, we can bring the research into clinical practice, but we have to manage the change process carefully and have a multidisciplinary team approach to the whole process from start to finish of a clinical audit trail. Auditing and monitoring clinical practice can be seen by some as threatening, but the reality is that bad practice or ineffective practice needs to be stopped and superseded by effective measures to ensure positive patient outcomes. If the evidence is available to support change, then so be it – we should strive to better the care we give to our patients on a continual basis.

Recap and recall

- Clinical guidelines are designed to help health professionals in their clinical decisions and to try and standardise care given to patients

- Clinical guidelines give recommendations on the action to be taken but they do not replace clinical judgement and experience. They do not always take into account individual variations in patients with a certain condition

- Clinical guidelines can be used in the education and training of health professionals and also to help patients and their carers to make informed choices about their care

- If used correctly, clinical guidelines can help to protect health professionals from litigation suits

- The NHS Centre for Review and Dissemination recommend that clinical guidelines have characteristics such as cost-effectiveness, reproducibility, reliability, representative development, clinical applicability, clinical flexibility, clarity, meticulous documentation, scheduled review and utilisation review

- Once a clinical guideline has been written and is ready for use, it has to be disseminated and implemented into clinical practice
- Potential advantages and disadvantages of clinical guidelines can be described in terms of effects on the patient, the health professional and the healthcare service. These three perspectives need to be considered in the development of the clinical guideline
- Clinical audit is the measurement of practice against agreed standards
- Clinical audit is a cyclical process which involves selecting the topic to review, agreeing the standards of best practice, defining the methodology, piloting the methods and collecting data, analysing and reporting of the results, making recommendations for change, implementing the change and monitoring this change and re-auditing
- A few terms may be confused with clinical audit. These include research, service evaluation and service improvement. You need to understand what the difference is between these separate processes
- To be effective clinical audit requires a multidisciplinary team approach, evidence-based standards, monitoring of practice and commitment to change from all concerned.

Key terms

Litigation The act or process of bringing or contesting a lawsuit.

Multidisciplinary team A team of healthcare professionals from different disciplines who work together to achieve a common aim.

Rates of morbidity The amount of suffering brought on from having a disease. This can be measured, for example, by quality-of-life scales or a level of disability.

Rates of mortality The number of deaths in a given period from a certain disease or condition.

Reliability A measure of the consistency and accuracy of data collection. A data collection instrument may be said to be unreliable if it generates different readings on repeated measurements at the same time of the same person. Low reliability can cause a research study to lack validity, but high reliability does not necessarily ensure validity.

Validity The extent to which data and its interpretation reflects the phenomenon under investigation without bias. Studies and instruments used to collect data are unlikely to be valid unless they are also reliable. Some qualitative researchers prefer to use terms such as credibility and trustworthiness to describe this concept.

Post-test

You might like to check your knowledge and understanding with these questions. You will find the correct answers at the end of the book.

1. What is a clinical guideline?

2. What is the overall aim of clinical guidelines?

3. List three positive aspects of clinical guidelines.

4. List three negative aspects of clinical guidelines.

5. Outline six characteristics of clinical guidelines.

6. Name the nine stages in the development and implementation of clinical guidelines.

7. What is clinical audit?

8. What are the stages in the clinical audit cycle?

9. What crucial factors are needed for clinical audit to be effective?

References and further reading

BTS/SIGN. (2010) *British Asthma Guidelines*. http://www.brit-thoracic.org.uk/ clinical-information/asthma/asthma-guidelines.aspx

Cookson, R., McDaid, D., Maynard, A. (2001) Wrong SIGN, NICE mess; is national guidance distorting allocation of resources? *British Medical Journal*, **323:** 743-5.

Department of Health. (1989) *Working for Patients*. London: HMSO.

Department of Health. (1996) *Promoting Clinical Effectiveness: a Framework for Action in and through the NHS*. Leeds: NHS Executive.

Duff, L.A., Kitson, A.L., Seers, K. (1996) Clinical guidelines; an introduction to their development and implementation. *Journal of Advanced Nursing*, **23:** 887-95.

Eccles, M., Grimshaw, J. (eds) (2000) *Clinical Guidelines from Conception to Use*. Oxon: Radcliffe Medical Press.

Field, M.J., Lohr, K.N. (1990) *Clinical Practice Guidelines: Directions for a New Program*. Washington: National Academies Press.

Grilli, R., Magrini, N., Penn, A. (2000) Practice guidelines developed by speciality societies; the need for critical appraisal. *Lancet*, **355:** 103-6.

Heffner, J.E. (1998) Does evidence-based medicine help the development of clinical practice guidelines? *Chest*, **113**(3): Suppl: 173S-8S.

Kayne, R.I. (1995) Creating practice guidelines; the dangers of over-reliance on expert judgment. *Journal of Law, Medicine and Ethics*, **23:** 62-4.

Mann, T. (1996) *Clinical Guidelines: Using Clinical Guidelines to Improve Patient Care in the NHS*. London: HMSO.

NHS Centre for Review and Dissemination. (1994) *Implementing Clinical Practice Guidelines*. Leeds: University of Leeds.

NICE. (2004) *The Guideline Development Process: an Overview for Stakeholders, the Public and the NHS*. London: NICE.

NICE/CHI. (2002) *Principles of Best Practice in Clinical Audit*. London: NICE.

Websites

Agency for healthcare research and quality
www.ahrq.gov

National electronic library for health guidelines database
www.nelh.nhs.uk/guidelines_database.asp

NICE
www.nice.org.uk

RCN clinical guidelines
www.rcn.org.uk/services/promote/clinical/clinical_guidelines.htm

Chapter 5

Change management in the implementation of evidence-based practice

AIMS

When you have read this chapter, you should understand:

- What change management is and what some of the theories and models for this are
- Considerations that need to be incorporated into any change process
- Barriers to change and how to alleviate them
- What professional, legal and ethical considerations need to be made when implementing evidence base into clinical practice

Introduction

So far we have discussed what evidence is, where it comes from and how to evaluate and critique it. The development and use of clinical guidelines has also been discussed with reference to evidence-based practice. The final part of this process is to implement it into clinical practice, to influence or change practice for the good of the patient and service user.

The process of implementation is a team effort and therefore is dependent on the team and the culture that exists within the organisation. Changing practice requires energy, motivation and support from others and these need to be sustained over a period of time; as discussed in the previous chapter around clinical audit.

There are several key considerations when thinking about implementing evidence base into practice. Firstly, a topic area needs to be established, and of most importance is that there is a positive patient benefit. The primary aim of evidence-based practice has been defined as identification and application of 'the most efficacious interventions to maximise the quality and quantity of life for individual patients' (Sackett *et al.*, 1996: p. 4). However, it is not always enough that the literature shows positive benefits for patients – healthcare professionals need to be persuaded that any change will be manageable for them and that the resources needed are already available.

It can be argued that the definition of evidence-based practice given above can be equally applied to the traditional decision-making that goes on by healthcare professionals in clinical practice during their normal duties of work, where the healthcare professionals' knowledge of the literature and clinical experience and expertise are used to meet patients' needs.

ACTIVITY 5.1

Can you think of any changes that have been made in your clinical area? If so, was this because of new evidence that had emerged on the topic area or was it because of other reasons such as cost cuts?

....

....

....

Change management in the NHS

The need for change in the health service is widely recognised by health professionals, the government and the public. Evidence should constantly be reviewed and practices questioned to ensure that they are the 'best way' and that true quality care is constantly strived for by all concerned in the health service. *The NHS Plan* (Department of Health, 2000) brought about a fundamental change in the thinking and ways of delivering care and, in addition, sustaining quality was highlighted alongside this. In the White Paper *A First Class Service* (Department of Health, 1998), the **NCCSDO** was commissioned to undertake a review of the evidence around the topic area of change management. From this it was concluded that there was evidence available on what works and what does not in terms of change within the health service. It was concluded that the NHS must make use of this evidence to drive forward with developing and maintaining a quality service for all.

Sometimes, change can be deliberate, as a product of conscious reasoning and actions. This is referred to as planned change, and on occasion can occur due to assumptions made by managers, rather than evidence base. I am sure that some of us can relate to this situation. On the other hand, change sometimes unfolds in a more spontaneous and unplanned way. This is called emergent change, an example of which could be change owing to external factors such as the economic and political climate (Upton and Brookes, 1995). These two distinct forms of change highlight two important aspects to consider when managing any change in the health service, these being:

1. The need to identify, explore and, if necessary, challenge the assumptions that underlie managerial decisions.

2. The ability to understand the organisational change as a process that can be facilitated by perceptive and insightful planning and analysis and a sensitive implementation phase.

Change can also be understood in relation to its extent and scope. Ackerman (1997) has distinguished between three types of change: developmental, transitional and transformational.

1. Developmental change may be either planned or emergent. It is change that should enhance or correct existing aspects of an organisation and often focuses on the improvement of skills or processes, so is very relevant to the health service in this aspect for obvious reasons.

2. Transitional change seeks to achieve a known desired state that is different from the existing one. It is episodic, planned or radical – this may not sometimes be suited to the health service, as radical change can bring about many barriers from both staff and patients. The model of transitional change has its origins in the work of Lewin (1951), who conceptualised change as a three-stage process involving unfreezing the existing organisational equilibrium, moving to a new position and refreezing in a new position. This sounds very neat and simple, but in reality I am sure you can imagine that this is not the case, especially in a complex organisation like the health service.

3. Transformational change is rather radical in nature. It requires a shift in assumptions made by the organisation and its members. Transformation can result in an organisation that differs significantly in terms of structure, processes, culture and strategy. It may, therefore, result in the creation of an organisation that operates in developmental mode, which is one that continuously learns, adapts and improves. This could be said for the health service in some aspects of its organisation and delivery of objectives and patient outcomes.

ACTIVITY 5.2

Now that you have read some of the models and approaches to change in organisations, which do you think would be the most appropriate to your organisation and area of practice and why? This will help you to understand further the complex thought processes that go on when planning any change in practice.

....

....

....

....

Many approaches to organisational change found in the literature give the impression that change is a rational, controlled and orderly process. In practice, it can be chaotic, involving shifts in goals and some unexpected occurrences along the way, even when planning has preceded the change. This is especially so in the NHS, which is a very complex organisation with multiple factors to consider.

A further approach in change management to consider is the 'systems thinking approach'. This approach originated in the 1920s and grew out of an observation that there were many aspects of organisations that scientific analysis could not explore. Scientific method breaks things down into constituent parts and explores them individually. Systems thinking explores the properties that exist once the parts have been combined into a whole.

In terms of understanding organisations, systems thinking suggests that issues, events, forces and incidents should not be viewed as isolated phenomena, but seen as interconnected, interdependent components of a complex entity, which is very relevant to the health service. Applied to change management, the systems thinking approach highlights the following:

1. A system is made up of related and interdependent parts, so that any system must be viewed as a whole.

2. A system cannot be viewed in isolation from the environment.

3. A system that is in equilibrium will change only if some type of energy is applied.

4. Players within a system have a view of that system's function and purpose, and players' views may be very different from each others'.

Within the NHS the term 'whole systems thinking' is now routinely used by managers and clinicians. This widespread usage reflects an increase in:

1. Awareness of the multifactorial issues involved in healthcare, which mean that complex health and social patterns lie beyond the ability of any one practitioner, team or agency to 'fix'.

2. Interest in designing, planning and managing organisations as living, independent systems, committed to providing 'seamless' care for patients.

3. Use of large group interventions to bring together the perspectives of a broad range of stakeholders across a wide system.

Pollitt (1993) and Dawson (1999) suggest that the NHS is characterised by three defining features:

1. Range and diversity of **stakeholders**.
2. Complex ownership and resourcing arrangements.
3. **Professional autonomy** of many of its staff.

The NHS is a large organisation employing people with a wide range of talents, perspectives and passions. It is a complex organisation, with many different **cultures** and norms arising from a number of factors, including:

1. Different socialisation processes of professions.
2. Different needs and expectations of different client groups.
3. Different histories of different institutions.
4. Local priorities, resource allocation and performance management.

The complexity is a result of the very socialisation that has produced so many advances in healthcare. The specialisation also leads to a high degree of interdependence between practitioners and between practitioners and process. The interdependence and continuing technical and organisational advances mean that services and organisations within the NHS are dynamic as well as complex.

Meeting organisational change in the NHS therefore involves working with:

1. Changing pressures in the environment.
2. Multiple stakeholders within and outside the organisation.
3. Changing technologies available to those stakeholders.
4. Complex organisations in which individuals and teams are interdependent, i.e. they can only achieve their objectives by relying on other people seeking to achieve different objectives.
5. People who have experience of change interventions that have had unforeseen or unintended consequences.

It is also important to remember that cause and effect relationships may not be easily apparent, and that an intervention in any part of a healthcare organisation will have outcomes in many others, not all of them anticipated and not all of them desirable. The fact that change can lead to unanticipated and, indeed, dysfunctional consequences has been highlighted. For all these reasons change in the NHS is never likely to be straightforward and linear. Proposed change needs to offer benefits of interest to frontline staff and the approach needs to be interactive and to relate research clearly to current practice (Ywye and McClenahan, 2000).

SWOT analysis

SWOT is an acronym for examining an organisation's (or individual's) Strengths, Weaknesses, Opportunities and Threats, and using the result to identify priorities for action (Ansoff, 1965). The main principle underlying SWOT is that internal and external factors must be considered simultaneously when identifying aspects of an organisation that need to be changed. Strengths and weaknesses are internal to the organisation, while opportunities and threats are external.

For strengths and weaknesses the questions asked are:

1. What are the consequences of this?

2. Do they help or hinder us in achieving our missions?

3. If the factor helps in achieving the mission/aim, then it is a strength. If it is a hindrance then it is a weakness.

4. What are the causes of this strength/weakness?

For opportunities and threats the questions are slightly different:

1. What impact is this likely to have on us? Will it help or hinder us in achieving our missions? Again, only if the opportunity helps the team achieve the mission can it be considered such; even if it causes the world to be a nicer place, but fails to impact on the team's ability to achieve its mission, it will not be an opportunity for these purposes.

2. What must we do to respond to this opportunity?

The answers are then analysed, paying particular attention to the causes of the strengths and weaknesses and to the responses required to the opportunities and threats. Common threads are linked together into a set of priorities for the team to address.

Barriers to change

Reasons for resisting change in the NHS as well as any other organisation can include:

1. Loss of control or fear of loss of control
2. Too much uncertainty
3. Confusion from misunderstanding or from incorrect information given
4. Loss of face
5. Concerns about competence in a new context
6. Increased workload
7. Change fatigue
8. The view that costs outweigh benefits
9. Past resentments
10. Real threats.

In healthcare settings, a range of specific interventions have been used to try to change individual clinicians' behaviour. These include:

1. Educational outreach
2. Audit and feedback
3. Access to local opinion leaders
4. Patient-specific reminders
5. Continuing professional development (CPD)
6. Dissemination of guidelines.

Their effectiveness in securing change in clinical behaviour may provide some insights for those managing change in a wider context throughout the organisation. Managers need to accept that people in a system see things differently. There is a need, therefore, for managers to recognise this difference and respond creatively to work towards mutual trust and understanding based on transparency and honesty.

Level of change

Change can take place at many different levels in the NHS. This can be broadly classified as the macro and micro levels of healthcare. Macro changes can be classified as those at a national or strategic level, whereas micro change is more individualised, area/ward-based, or concerning change to individual attitudes and behaviours.

Evidence-based healthcare plays a part at both macro and micro levels. It is important that healthcare practitioners clarify at the outset the level at which they are operating, the types of innovation that are appropriate and feasible at that level, and the systems, individuals and groups that they are likely and unlikely to be able to influence.

Effective change is most likely to occur where it is focused on problem-solving and practice-based activities over which healthcare professionals have some control or influence. It is less likely to occur with activities that are more remote from the healthcare professional's day-to-day concerns and responsibilities (Davies *et al.*, 1995; Kitson *et al.*, 1998).

Change models

Bringing about change in healthcare practice is not straightforward and there are no panaceas or magic bullets for doing this. There are many models, but Lomas (1993) has identified three such models for the transfer of evidence into clinical and professional practice. These are:

1. *Passive diffusion model*: this assumes that healthcare professionals read or hear about research evidence and then adopt this in their practice. In the diffusion model, CPD is assumed to play a key role. However, the evidence from systematic reviews suggests that widely used CPD delivery methods, such as conferences, have little direct impact on improving professional practice (Davies *et al.*, 1995).

2. *Active dissemination model*: this is considered more effective than the model described above. It requires purposive action to promote knowledge and evidence to already busy healthcare professionals; this might include action by the Cochrane collaboration and journals, seminars and workshops. It is important to recognise that individuals are not simply sponges, soaking up new information without filtering or processing. Rather, new knowledge is shaped by the learner's pre-existing knowledge and experience.

3. *Coordinated implementation model*: in this model patients and community interest groups, healthcare administrators and public and clinical policy-makers are key players in bringing about effective change. Prompting effective change involves product champions from each of these groups, who can prepare locally led analysis of what needs to be done and what measures need to be taken to do this. This requires a shift in culture from research into practice, where evidence is generated by people separated from those in day-to-day practice, to research in practice, in which evidence generation and professional practice are much more closely connected (Nutley *et al.*, 2003).

Evidence from successful change in practice suggests that this requires an environment that is genuinely collaborative, cooperative, democratic, non-hierarchical and which involves all stakeholder groups. There needs to be ownership of the area where change is indicated and also of the change process. Some of these conditions are not always present in the healthcare setting.

Strategies to help implement evidence-based change

It is worth considering some of the strategies that can be used to create change in the health service. Needham (2000) identifies six such strategies:

1. Passive dissemination – such as publishing research findings, sending policy documents and guidelines to practitioners and managers.

2. Education – such as running conferences or workshops about new developments.

3. Marketing – actively promoting change to targeted groups or individuals who have the power to initiate these changes.

4. Mass media – creating a widespread awareness of the potential benefits of change and so creating informal pressure for its implementation.

5. Performance management – assessing the performance of a group or an individual and giving feedback.

6. Incentives and rewards – such as promotion or pay awards, based on the achievement of targets.

ACTIVITY 5.3

In your experience, or in your view, which strategy would be the most effective and why? Which would be the least effective and why? Think about this in relation to your own area of clinical practice or work.

....

....

....

....

....

....

Changing personal practice

Creating a genuine, long-lasting change in the practice of a group of healthcare professionals is daunting and difficult for even the most experienced practitioner. However, any healthcare professional has true potential to change their personal practice to some degree, if they want to. These changes need to be evidence-based, and the skills of evaluating the evidence base are essential. But what happens if there is little or no identifiable evidence to support the intended change? This can be frustrating.

One way of resolving this is through 'practitioner inquiry'. Shaw (2005: p. 1232) describes practitioner inquiry as evaluation research, development or more general inquiry that is small scale, local, grounded and carried out by professionals who directly deliver these services. In a nutshell, it is a form of inquiry taken on by healthcare professionals about their own area of practice, with an aim to explore, explain and maybe alter practice to ensure it is as effective as possible. One problem with this is that the practitioner can produce bias in their evaluation, especially if their role or job depends on this. Is that then the true implementation of evidence base into practice?

Incorporating patients' values

We have spoken about change and mentioned healthcare professionals, administrators and managers, but who does this change in practice ultimately affect? The answer is the patients and the users of the service. This can be a very complicated process, which involves healthcare professionals sharing the evidence with patients whilst also attempting to understand the patients' values and views and understanding. This can be extremely variable. Unfortunately, communicating evidence about benefits and harms to patients in a way that allows them to understand their choices and incorporate their preferences and values may be almost impossible at times, and trying to understand their individual values is even more complex.

Patients often have preferences not only about the outcomes, but also about the decision-making process. These preferences can vary and the patient's desired level of involvement should determine how the healthcare professional approaches this scenario. A shared decision-making approach is the approach most used and is the most effective. To do this certain decision-making aids need to be provided, such as written information on the condition, benefits, harms and options; probabilities of benefits and harms and balanced stories of others' experience or outcomes.

The most common way of incorporating patients' views into the decision-making process about changing practice will be through patient organisations and groups such as PALS (Patient Advice and Liaison Services) and the expert patient forums.

Healthcare professionals, legal and professional aspects of incorporating evidence-based change in the health service

Professional self-regulation allows health professionals to set their own standards of professional practice, conduct and discipline. In 2003, the Council of Healthcare Regulatory Excellence was created following some major cases of misconduct, as a statutory overarching body covering all of the UK. Its role is to promote best practice and consistency in regulation of healthcare professionals by the regulatory bodies of the General Medical Council (GMC), the Nursing and Midwifery Council (NMC) and the Health Professions Council (HPC). These regulatory bodies set standards and ensure that they keep up to date with change in clinical practice and expectations of the healthcare professions. They also function to maintain the trust of the public at large and, to achieve this, the healthcare professions have to be openly accountable for the standards they set and the way these are enforced.

The standards are documented in the profession's code of conduct or code of practice, which provides guidelines and requirements that all members of the profession are expected to follow. Characteristically these codes give guidance, in the form of principles regarding issues such as consent, confidentiality, autonomy, advocacy and duty of care. Of all these principles, one of the most significant in terms of evidence-based practice is that of informed consent.

As evidence-based practice has developed, the related concept of evidence-based choice has also developed, which will inevitably impact on the way informed consent is obtained. When appraising the best available evidence to provide patients with evidence-based information, healthcare professionals should therefore weigh up the advantages and disadvantages to the patients beforehand and be open and honest about these. It has been shown that giving evidence to patients does alter patients' views and decisions and hence enhances informed consent in evidence-based practice.

As healthcare professionals we have a duty of care and can be sued for negligence if we do not abide by the evidence supplied to us, to enable the best evidence-based care to be given. Healthcare professionals also have an obligation to ensure that patients receive information that is evidence-based and written in a format to allow informed consent to take place.

ACTIVITY 5.4

Think about the information that you regularly give out to your patients, or that you see being given out to patients. Does it incorporate research-based information? Does the information given allow patients to make an informed choice? Can you think how some of this information may be improved?

....

....

....

....

....

Conclusion

As a final point, many reading this book are probably students who are yet to qualify. It is a known fact that nurses and other healthcare professionals must be responsible and accountable for keeping their own knowledge and skills up to date through continued professional development and lifelong learning. They must use evaluation, supervision and appraisal to improve their performance and to enhance the safety and quality of care and service delivery.

You must also recognise the limits of your own competence and knowledge. You must reflect on your own practice and seek advice from, or refer to, other professionals where necessary.

It must also be recognised and appreciated that, as newly qualified health professionals, you should not be expected suddenly to take on this element of your role. You have many other new elements of your role to learn. Being qualified is very different from being a student and it takes time to gain a grounding in your new area and understand your new role. Once settled, then start to evaluate the evidence put forward in your area of practice.

Recap and recall

- Changing practice requires energy, motivation and support from others and these need to be sustained over a period of time
- When implementing evidence base into practice, a topic area needs to be established, which has benefits of positive patient outcomes
- It can be argued that evidence-based practice can be equally applied to the traditional decision-making that goes on by healthcare professionals in clinical practice during their normal duties of work
- Planned change is a product of conscious reasoning and actions
- Emergent change is that which unfolds in a more spontaneous and unplanned way

- Developmental change may be either planned or emergent and often focuses on changing or enhancing an existing aspect of an organisation

- Transitional change requires a shift in assumptions made by the organisation and its members. It can result in an organisation that differs in terms of structure, processes, culture and strategy

- Systems thinking approach suggests that issues, events, forces and incidents should not be viewed as isolated phenomena, but seen as interconnected, interdependent components of a complete entity

- Within the NHS the term 'whole systems approach' is routinely used

- SWOT analysis is an acronym for examining organisations or individuals, which results in the identification of priorities for action

- Barriers to change can include loss of control or fear of loss of control, too much uncertainty, confusion and misunderstanding, loss of face, increased workload, the view that costs outweigh the benefits, and past experiences and resentments

- In the NHS a range of interventions is used to try to change individual clinician's behaviour, such as education, audit and feedback, patient-specific reminders and dissemination of guidelines

- The level at which change takes place is either macro (national or strategic) or micro (local, individual or area/ward-based)

- Models of change include the passive diffusion model, the active dissemination model and the coordinated implementation model

- Strategies to help implement evidence-based change include passive dissemination, education, marketing, mass media, performance management and incentives and rewards

- 'Practitioner inquiry' is a form of inquiry taken on by healthcare professionals about their own area of practice, with the aim of exploring, explaining and maybe altering practice to ensure it is as effective as possible

- Patients often have preferences, not only about the outcomes, but also about the decision-making process. A shared decision-making process is therefore essential

- The most important element of professional responsibilities in evidence-based practice is informed consent. To achieve this patients must be provided with information and literature to aid their understanding about the decision they are to take.

Key terms

Culture of an organisation Describes the specific collection of values and norms that are shared by people and groups in an organisation that control the way they interact with each other and with stakeholders outside the organisation.

NCCSDO National Coordinating Centre for NHS Service Delivery and Organisation.

Professional autonomy The quality or state of being independent and self-directing, especially in making decisions and enabling professionals to exercise judgement as they see fit during the performance of their job.

Stakeholders Groups of individuals whose support for the organisation keeps it going. Without this the organisation would not exist. For example, stakeholders for the NHS include the government, trust chairs, management, employees, unions, suppliers, commissioners, etc.

Post-test

You might like to check your knowledge and understanding with these questions. You will find the correct answers at the end of the book.

1. Can you give a definition of change management?

2. Name three models of change.

3. What is the difference between transitional and transformational change?

4. Name three considerations that need to be implemented in any change process in the health service.

5. Name five barriers to change that may occur.

6. Name three strategies that may help to relieve any barriers to change.

7. Why is it important to give appropriate information to patients to aid them in their decision-making process?

References and further reading

Ackerman, L. (1997) Developmental transitions or transformation: the question of change in organisations. In: D. Van Eynde, J. Hay, D. Van Eynde (eds) *Organisational Development Classics*. San Francisco: Jossey Bass.

Ackoff, R.L. (1970) *Redesigning the Future: a Systems Approach to Societal Problems*. New York: Wiley.

Ansoff, H.I. (1965) *Corporate Strategy: an Analytic Approach to Business Policy for Growth and Expansion*. London: McGraw Hill.

Davies, D.A., Thomson, M.A., Oxman, A.D. (1995) Changing physician performance: a systematic review of the effect of continuing medical education. *Journal of the American Medical Society*, **274**(9): 700-5.

Dawson, S. (1999) Managing, organising and performing in health care: what do we know and how do we learn? In: A. Mark., S. Dopson (eds) *Organisational Behaviour in Healthcare*. London: Macmillan.

Department of Health. (1998) *A First Class Service*. London: HMSO.

Department of Health. (2000) *The NHS Plan: a Plan for Investment, a Plan for Reform*. London: HMSO.

Grol, R.C. (1997) Beliefs and evidence in changing clinical practice. *British Medical Journal*, **315**: 418-21.

Kitson, A., Harvey, G., MacCormack, B. (1998) Enabling the implementation of evidence-based practice: a conceptual framework. *Quality in Health Care*, **7**: 149-58.

Lewin, K. (1951) *Field Theory in Social Science*. New York: Harper Row.

Lomas, R. (1993) Change models. In: J. Rycroft-Malone, T. Bucknall (eds) (2010). *Models and Frameworks for Implementing Evidence Based Practice: Linking Evidence to Action*. London: Wiley-Blackwell.

Needham, G. (2000) Research and practice: making a difference. In: R. Gomm, C. Davies (eds) *Using Evidence in Health and Social Care*. London: Sage.

Newman, M., Papadopoulos, I., Sigsworth, J. (1998) Barriers to evidence based practice. *Clinical Effectiveness in Nursing*, **2**: 11-20.

NHS Centre of Review and Dissemination. (1999) Getting evidence into practice. *Effective Health Care*, **5**: 1.

Nutley, S., Walter, I., Davies, H.T. (2003) From knowing to doing: a framework for understanding the evidence-into-practice agenda. *Evaluation*, **9**(2): 125-48.

Pollitt, C. (1993) The struggle for quality: the case of the NHS. *Policy and Politics*, **21**(3): 161-70.

Popper, K. (1972) *Objective Knowledge*. Oxford: Oxford University Press.

Rycroft-Malone, J., Harvey, G., Seers, K. (2004) An explanation of the factors that influence the implementation of evidence into practice. *Journal of Clinical Nursing*, **13**(8): 913-24.

Sackett, D.L., Richardson, W.S., Rosenburg, W. (1996) *Evidence Based Medicine: how to Practice and Teach Evidence Based Medicine*. New York: Churchill Livingstone.

Shaw, I. (2005) Practitioner research: evidence or critique? *British Journal of Social Work*, **35**: 1231-48.

Thompson, C. (2003) Clinical experience as evidence in evidence based practice. *Journal of Advanced Nursing*, **43**(3): 230-7.

Upton, T., Brookes, B. (1995) *Managing Change in the NHS*. London: Kogan Page.

Ywye, L., McClenahan, T. (2000) *Getting Better with Evidence: Experience of Putting Evidence into Practice*. London: Kings Fund.

Answers to post-test questions

Chapter 1

1. The stages of the research process are formation of the topic area, defining the hypothesis, justification of why the research needs to be done, defining the methodology, pilot study, redefining the methodology if necessary, gathering the data, analysis of data, discussion of results, recommendations to clinical practice and future research.

2. Differences between qualitative and quantitative research include qualitative research aims to gather an in-depth understanding of human behaviour, the data is narrative and is analysed for themes and understanding. Quantitative research is about numbers. Data is numerical and is analysed with statistical techniques.

3. Methodologies used in qualitative research include grounded theory, phenomenology, ethnography and action research.

4. Methodologies used in quantitative research include randomised controlled trials, cohort or case studies and cross-sectional or survey studies.

5. Qualitative research generates narrative data.

6. Quantitative research produces numerical data.

Chapter 2

1. Evidence is information from research, professional experience, clinical experience, patients and carers, which is used to base our decisions on in clinical practice. Sources of evidence can come from research studies, professional and clinical experience and knowledge.

2. Evidence-based practice is an approach to decision-making in which the clinician uses the best evidence available, in consultation with the patient, to decide upon the option that suits the patient best.

3. The five stages of evidence-based practice are defining the question, finding the evidence, appraisal of the evidence, acting on the evidence, evaluation and reflection on the results.

4. Useful online databases are MEDLINE, PubMed and CINAHL.

5. The key areas to reflect upon in evidence-based practice are that you are asking an appropriate question, that you have searched the most appropriate databases for the evidence, that an appropriate tool has been used to appraise the literature and that, when you have appraised the evidence and come to act upon it in terms of clinical practice, it is a multidisciplinary team process.

6. Systematic reviews and meta-analyses are ranked first in the hierarchy of evidence.

7. Views of colleagues and peers are ranked last in the hierarchy of evidence.

Chapter 3

1. Clinical effectiveness is all about achieving improved outcomes of care.

2. Clinical governance is a framework through which NHS organisations are accountable for continuously improving the quality of their services and safeguarding high standards of care by creating an environment in which excellence in clinical care can flourish.

3. Evidence-based practice is needed to ensure that quality of care and positive patient outcomes are developed and maintained. This is the objective/aim of clinical governance.

4. Components of clinical governance include audit, clinical effectiveness, risk management, research and development, education and training and CPD, staffing and staff development, openness and patient involvement.

5. The PEST framework can be used to help implement change. The factors to be considered include political factors, economic factors, technological factors and social factors.

6. Evidence is important to quality care because without good-quality evidence we would not see how things can be done differently to

achieve further quality outcomes in patient care. We would never change from how we have always done things and things move on so quickly in healthcare that we would soon be out of date and dangerous in our clinical practice.

Chapter 4

1. A clinical guideline is a systematically developed statement to assist practitioner decisions about appropriate healthcare for specific clinical conditions.

2. The overall aim of clinical guidelines is to improve the quality of care. This is done by providing the evidence and thus standardising care to some degree. They are designed to help healthcare professionals in their work. They are not there to replace clinical judgement and expertise.

3. Positive aspects of clinical guidelines include: they are evidence-based, improve consistency of care if used appropriately, can draw attention to under-recognised health problems, help in clinical decision-making and can draw attention to wasteful and dangerous practices. They can identify gaps in the evidence base where research can then be focused, they can protect the healthcare professional against litigation if used correctly, improve efficiency through standardisation, optimise value for money and can increase public confidence.

4. Negative aspects of clinical guidelines include the fact that the recommendations in them may be wrong, they may lack evidence in an area which affects the development of the guideline, not all patients fit the blanket recommendations given by the guidelines and lay versions can be inappropriately worded and lead to confusion.

5. Characteristics of guidelines include: validity, cost-effectiveness, reproducibility, reliability, representative development, clinical applicability, clinical flexibility, clarity, meticulous documentation, scheduled review and utilisation review.

6. The nine stages in the development and implementation of guidelines include: selection of the guideline topic, composition of the guideline development group, defining the scope of the

guideline, systematic literature review, formation of recommendations, consultation and peer review, presentation and dissemination, local implementation, audit and review.

7. Clinical audit is a quality improvement process that seeks to improve patient care and outcomes through systematic review of care against explicit criteria and the implementation of change.

8. The stages of clinical audit are selection of topic, agree standards of best practice, define methodology, pilot and data collection, analysis and reporting, make recommendations, implement change, re-audit.

9. The crucial factors needed for clinical audit to be effective are evidence-based standards, a multidisciplinary approach, monitoring of practice and commitment to change.

Chapter 5

1. Change management is about taking the evidence to drive forward and develop the health service to maintain a quality service for all.

2. Three models of change are the passive diffusion model, the active dissemination model and the coordinated implementation model.

3. Transitional change seeks to achieve a known desired state that is different from the existing one. Transformational change is more radical and requires a shift in assumptions made by the organisation and its members.

4. Three considerations that need to be implemented in any change process in the health service are: the need to identify, explore and, if necessary, challenge the assumptions that underlie managerial decision-making, being able to understand the organisational change as a process that can be facilitated by perceptive and insightful planning and analysis and a sensitive implementation phase, and an awareness of the multifactorial issues involved in healthcare.

5. Barriers to change include: loss of control or fear of loss of control, too much uncertainty, confusion from misunderstanding or from incorrect information given, loss of face, concerns about competence in a new context, increased workload, change fatigue,

the view that costs outweigh benefits, past resentments and real threats.

6. Strategies for relieving barriers to change include: educational outreach, audit and feedback, access to local opinion leaders, patient-specific reminders, CPD and dissemination of guidelines.

7. Appropriate information should be given to patients to aid their decision-making process. Because the aim is to have a shared decision-making process, there is a need to give accurate information to help patients form their views and opinions, there is a need to understand patients' values and views and understanding to aid effective service development. Patients often have views about the process as well as the outcomes. Accurate information will aid this.

Index

Note: definitions of **key terms** are indicated by **bold page numbers**